RSI, Repetitive Strain Injury caused by electronic gadgets, laptops, PC's and mobile phones.

Neck Pain? Shoulder Pain? Wrist Pain? Thumb Pain? It could be RSI, Repetitive Strain Injury.

by

Lucy Rudford

ALL RIGHTS RESERVED. This book contains material protected under International and Federal Copyright Laws and Treaties.

Any unauthorized reprint or use of this material is strictly prohibited. No part of this book may be reproduced or transmitted in any form or by any means, electronic, mechanical or otherwise, including photocopying or recording, or by any information storage and retrieval system without express written permission from the author.

Copyrighted © 2015

Published by IMB Publishing

Table of Contents

Table of Contents 3

Acknowledgments 4

Foreword by the Author. 5

Chapter 1. Is this Your Future? 8

Chapter 2. Repetitive Strain Injury: An Overview 14

Chapter 3. Treatment of RSIs 30

Chapter 4. Coping with a Repetitive Strain Injury 41

Chapter 5. Preventing Repetitive Strain Injuries 58

Chapter 6. Risk Assessment 76

Chapter 7. Dangers of Laptops 82

Chapter 8. Cell Phones, Video Games and Other Hand Held Devices ... 89

Chapter 9. RSI Concerns for Children and Teenagers 94

Chapter 10. RSIs in the Workplace 107

Chapter 11. Relevant Regulations 120

Chapter 12. Conclusion 124

Chapter 13. Stretchers and Exercises 126

Vendors of Equipment and Software for RSI Prevention 132

Acknowledgments

Thanks to my mum for being such a great mum. Even though she works long hours, she always has time to listen and help me. Her office door is always open to my sibling and I. She was the inspiration for this book.

In addition, my dad always supports mum and us kids in whatever we do. He's always there with an encouraging word and an understanding heart. I especially thank him for taking the time to read this book and offer his valuable suggestions on how to make it better.

Without my brothers and sisters, especially my amazing twin sister, to make me laugh, I would never have been able to complete this project.

I also want to thank all the people who generously shared their personal experiences about living with repetitive strain injuries. I've learned so much from them and appreciate their openness and honesty. The stories and quotes in the book (the ones that are not attributed to specific sources) are based on what these people with RSIs told me.

Thanks goes to all the professionals in the field that I spoke to whose experience and knowledge helped me understand the big problem Repetitive Strain Injury is in our electronic society.

My friends not only inspired this book, they also told me their stories and encouraged me to write. May they be safe and healthy and live well.

A special thank you to Lasun Sosanya, an Extended Scoop Physiotherapist, who is a friend of the family. To make sure that all the information in this book is correct, I have asked him to read this book and to approve all the information and exercises in this book.

Foreword by the Author.

I am 19 years old and I consider myself a hard working student. I am not a doctor but I did ask a specialist in the field to read this book for me. All the knowledge I have about RSI is gathered by studying the subject, speaking to sufferers and talking to specialists.

I was just a regular teenager, with lots of friends I kept in touch with by texting. But then my thumbs started to hurt. It was a strange feeling. At first I tried to ignore it, then I convinced myself it would go away. But it didn't go away--the pain kept getting worse.

One day I mentioned my hurting sore thumbs to my friends. I felt a little silly about it, but most of them had their own complaints. Thumbs, wrists, arms—they all had pain somewhere. When we compared notes, we realized something strange was going on and we 'd better deal with it.

Then, I went to the doctor and he told me that I could have repetitive strain injury, or RSI. He thought it was because of all the texting I do. The doctor told me it's becoming an epidemic amongst young people. He also told me it's very serious and could affect my whole life if I didn't take care of it now.

I was stunned. Surely at the age of 19, I couldn't possible have RSI? I didn't want to end up suffering like my mum, but how could I give up texting? I decided I would help to prevent RSIs in young people. I talked to my friends and urged them to take it all seriously. Teenagers don't want to hear about the future, but I kept telling them that if they didn't pay attention now they may not be able to work when they get older or even enjoy life in different ways.

So I decided to write a book to make more people, especially young people, aware of the dangers of the electronic devices we love so much. I wanted to get the message across that you don't have to give up your cell phones , computers and game boys, but you do have to make changes now or you are going to pay for it later.

I learned so much researching and writing this book. What's different about this book is that it covers issues for young people and for adults. It focuses on RSIs in the technological environment of the 21st Century.

According to an extended scope physiotherapist I have spoken to, when today's youngsters will be 40 it will already be too late and nothing but surgery will help RSI. Surgery of course cannot always be done in certain cases therefore suffering the rest of your life is the only option left. That is just scary stuff.

Anyone who uses a computer, laptop, tablet, game console or a mobile phone regularly is at risk and should know about RSI. Unfortunately most people do not understand what RSI is and are uninformed therefore they do not realise how serious it can be.

This book is intended to educate mostly youngsters about RSI and to provide useful suggestions for prevention and treatment. It is my aim to make young as well as older people aware of the potential dangers of all the electronic gadgets that we all so love.

Imagine this worse but at the same time very realistic scenario: You've been studying really hard and you are looking forward to a successful career ahead of you. As a student, you have spent a lot of time texting and using laptops and you have been ignoring the pains in your thumb and neck. You finally got your first job with a very good chance to get promoted within a few months and end up in your DREAM job. After 2 months your dreams are shattered as you have been told you have RSI and you are strongly advised not to sit on the computer any longer or you might end up in a wheelchair! You have to give up your job, your career and your dreams and all that because you did not pay attention to your first symptoms of RSI! Surely you would do it differently next time if you could change things.

There are three things (all discussed further in the book) that I encourage absolutely everybody to do whilst texting, working on a pc, a laptop/tablet or playing on a game console:

* TAKE REGULAR BREAKS

* DO REGULAR EXERCISES e.g. stretch your neck, arms and back as described further in this book.

* MAKE SURE YOU ARE SITTING IN THE CORRECT POSITION whilst on your PC or laptop (not on your bed with your laptop on your lap) and if you can afford it, buy an ergonomic chair.

I hope that my book not only helps you to prevent RSI but also helps you to deal with it.

It is no joke, really, please take this seriously and look after your future health.

Don't ignore your symptoms as it really comes down to this one simple message:

ACT NOW

OR

SUFFER FOREVER!

Chapter 1. Is this Your Future?

1) Scary stories

Below you will find some quotes/stories from people that I spoke to or people that I found on forums.

These stories are INTENTIONALLY at the beginning of this book to encourage people to read the whole book. I realise that it is difficult to convince young people (and also older people) to read a whole book about RSI but perhaps these stories do make you understand how bad RSI can get if you if you DON'T ACT NOW.

Some of the stories are repeated in the book simply because repetition is good for remembering. Other stories that I list here are not repeated in the book.

A pupil's Story: *Four years ago I developed a repetitive strain injury in both hands, wrists, arms, shoulders and neck. The vagus nerve was affected and after 15 minutes of doing any kind of work with my arms - washing up, driving, writing, working on the computer - I was in tears from the sickening, deadly aching pain. The hospital physiotherapist told me I presented the most severe and extensive case she had ever seen and warned me I was unlikely to recover fully. I spent hundreds of pounds each month visiting chiropractors, osteopaths and massage therapists, and although they all provided some relief, nothing lasted. I began to wonder if I could ever work again. Source: www.stat.org.uk*

RSI- sufferer's story (my mum): *For the last 5 years I have been sitting on the computer almost non-stop as I am a full time internet marketer. When I work too long, without breaks, my neck hurts. When my neck doesn't hurt, I have a headache on top of my head. When I don't have a headache, I get pain shoots in my legs. When my legs are fine, my back hurts. When....surely you get the message. My doctor tells me I have to change my lifestyle or I will be in a wheelchair in 10 years time. I am only 52 and I want to have fun with my grandchildren! Guess that's not going to happen in a wheelchair unless I change my life NOW. I WILL! All this because I didn't take enough breaks whilst on the computer. I always thought that an office environment is a place with very low risk of injury. I was wrong!*

Chapter 1. Is This Your Future?

Believe me, I have learned the hard way. For years I sat working on my computer for hours and days in the wrong position, in the wrong chair, without any breaks. On some days, I would switch my computer on at 8am and work on it until 1am the next morning. My punishment for this: I have been diagnosed with cervical spondolysis (a non-curable condition) in my neck, with disc space between C5, C6 and C7 most affected. Want proof? Here it is. As I always like to prove what I say, here is a picture of my neck's x-ray and MRI scan. You can see on the first picture that the space between disc C5 and C6 is thinner than all the other spaces. The second picture shows a bulging disc pushing pressure on the spinal cord and its nerves fibers. Permanent nerve damage can be caused when a bulging disc in the neck is compressing a nerve for a long period of time.

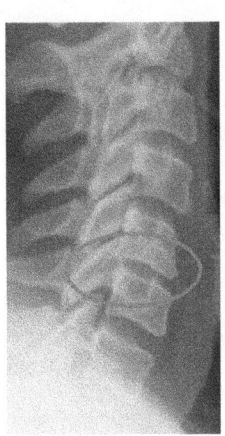 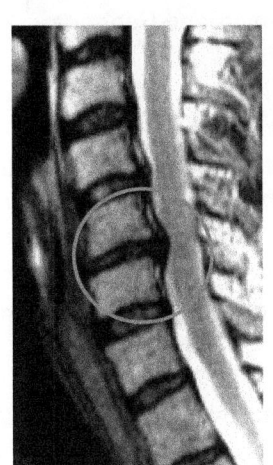

Now I cannot work on the computer as much as I would like to because when I do, my neck starts to hurt, my arm goes "dead" and I lose part of my grip and feelings in my arm. I now have two choices: work a long time and give myself pain or work less and have no pain. As health is more important than money I obviously choose to work fewer hours. I can still work long hours on the computer but certainly not as long as I would like to or I will make my condition worse. I am not telling you this out of self-pity as I am very happy with what I have achieved. I am telling you this so you won't make the same mistake! **Source: my mum!**

RSI-sufferer's story: *"I was rinsing off some spaghetti the other night and my fingers in the affected hand just let go of the colander - and the spaghetti landed in the sink. That was the end of another meal! I can't*

Chapter 1. Is This Your Future?

cut up my food properly or clean my teeth very well (although I have now bought a sonic wave toothbrush which helps with this task). When the pain and motor function is really bad, it's embarrassing to have to ask someone to unzip/unbutton my jeans or trousers so I can go to the loo, or having to ask my husband to cut up my food for me because I can't manage to do this simple task myself." Source: Watson, M. 2009. Investigating the experiences of people with RSI. http://etheses.qmu.ac.uk/

RSI-sufferer's story: " I am 19. After texting my boyfriend 10 times, my thumb starts hurting. When I sit on my bed using my laptop, my neck is painful. I am so glad my friend wrote this book as she made me realise I have to look after my health better. I now call my boyfriend instead of texting him." Source: my friend Georgina.

RSI-sufferer's story: " I am 20. I always "slouch" on my bed using my laptop, even when I study for my exams. Not any more after I've read what my twin sister wrote in her book. I constantly get lower back pains and now I realise it is because the way I "slouch" on my bed hanging forwards all the time. I am now sitting on my desk to use my laptop and I have installed software on my laptop (mum paid for it) that forces me to get up every 45 minutes to take a break. My lower back pains have stopped". Source: my adorable twin sis.

RSI-sufferers story: "At the moment, I have a pinched nerve in my neck, which causes quite extreme pain in my left shoulder, down my left arm and occasionally tingling in my fingers. It's not the first time, about 18 months ago I had the same, but on the other side - affecting my right arm!

"Painkillers help, obviously, but it looks like I am heading for some serious physiotherapy, not just to sort this particular issue out, but some of the other posture-related issues that playing some very heavy electric basses and guitars for 35 years have caused.

"Oh, and having also been an IT journalist, hunching over a keyboard for hours on end didn't help either, apparently. I'm really looking forward to the traction on my thoracic spine....

Chapter 1. Is This Your Future?

So, if you're young, correct your posture - and if you're not so young get checked out and take advice on correcting your posture - I wouldn't wish this pain on anyone." Source: Comment by Paul at the DIY Musician

RSI-sufferers story: "It pains me to write this – literally. My neck is crooked, one of my wrists feels like it has been trapped in a car door and there's a rapidly calcifying knot of nastiness lurking around my right shoulder blade... This is the price one pays for hammering a keyboard like Jerry Lee Lewis all day, every day for 15 years... Having blown all my wages on remedies, it seems the only real way to alleviate the ailment is to type less, which isn't easy when your entire working existence takes places electronically, you have book deadlines to meet and writing is all you can do. Source: Ben Myers in the Guardian 17 September 2010.

RSI-sufferers story: "Hi, I'm a 17 year old male. I have been having some joint pain in the last few weeks. Very recently, I noticed that my fingers were getting stiff. It started from the little finger in my left hand which was really stiff. When I bring any movements to the finger, it moves in a really edgy or a jerky way instead of the usual smooth movements. I sit in front of the computer for really long hours and I felt that this was the reason (RSI) for it. so I started taking frequent breaks but I don't think it helped that much. This problem has been getting worse from day to day. And yesterday I noticed the same thing happen in my right hand too. The little finger in both hands does not have limited range but movement (jerky). And this same problem is spreading to the other fingers as well. I'm feeling the same thing happen to my ring fingers too. No swelling has been observed but lack of movement, mild (sometimes severe in mornings) pain, loss of grip and mild pain on wrist. Symptoms are worse at times after I wake up from sleep where a huge portion of my fingers are stiff and difficultly to get a strong grip. The problems are also worse on colder days. Mostly while playing games, my left hand would be on the keyboard and my right hand on the mouse but since both hands are showing the same symptoms." Source: chatastrophy on Medhelp.org 10 August 2008 (Capitalization and punctuation added for ease of reading.)

RSI-sufferers story: "I was 22 and working as a legal secretary when I first felt pain in my arms. I ignored it, thinking or hoping it would go

Chapter 1. Is This Your Future?

away, and continued to work at my normal pace. I had recently changed jobs and didn't want to cause any problems. However, typing for six or seven hours a day I soon realised the pain was getting worse. I continued working for about six months then my employer put me off work. It got to the stage that I couldn't type more than a few minutes at a time and couldn't keep up with the workload. They didn't have any light duties for me nor did they want to re-instate me unless I could type as much as I had previously. In the end, they legally terminated my employment after I had been off work for six months." Source: RSI and Overuse Injury Association of the ACT

2) Scary pictures.
The truth hurts! These pictures show you what can happen to you if you don't take the messages in this book seriously. Don't think it won't happen to you as that is exactly what all the sufferers that I mentioned in this book thought. I will do everything I possibly can to make sure it won't happen to me though! Are you in with me? Sure hope so.

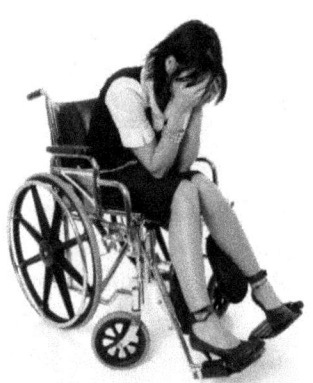

Do you want to end up like this by the age of 50? This is a very realistic outcome for children who start using modern electronic devices at the age of 8 and use them constantly every single day for many hours.

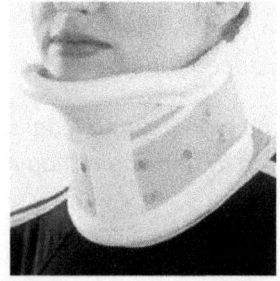

Chapter 1. Is This Your Future?

Or is this neck support collar what you want to be wearing when you are 40 because otherwise you have an unbearable pain in your neck because you've used your neck muscles in the wrong position for many years? Source: www.support4physio.com

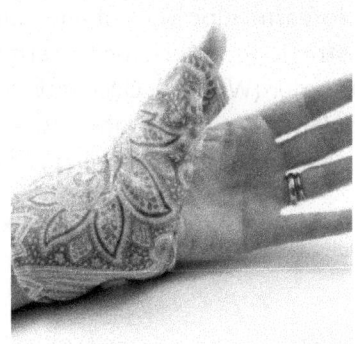

Source:www.theferriswheelshop.com

Or perhaps you want to wear a thumb wrap all the time for your texting thumb that hurts? They manufacturer these now in designs that are colourful and therefore appealing more to youngsters. Surely that must tell you that texting thumb is a huge problem.

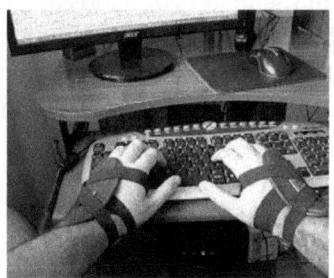

Or is this how you want to be typing when you're 30? Wearing gloves because without them you are simply in too much agony to type! Source: http://en.wikipedia.org/wiki/File:Luva.jpg

Chapter 2. Repetitive Strain Injury: An Overview

1. What is Repetitive Strain Injury (RSI)?

(RSI) refers to a group of injuries to the muscles, tendons, and nerves of the neck, shoulder, forearm, elbow, wrist and hands. RSIs cause pain, weakness and restrictions of movement. Terms such as Work-Related Upper Limb Disorder (WRULD), Occupational Overuse Syndrome (OOS), Cumulative Trauma Disorder (CTD), and Musculoskeletal Disorder (MSD) refer to similar groups of conditions.

Diagnoses like Fibromyalgia Syndrome (FMS) Reflex Sympathetic Hystrophy(RSD) and Chronic Fatigue Syndrome(CFS) are also family of RSI.

RSIs are serious and painful conditions, often debilitating and permanent. People who are severely injured cannot use their hands at all—not for computer work, feeding themselves, driving or turning the pages of a book. RSI is not a mental illness. The pain is not in our heads- the pain is very real. RSI is a result from overusing the hands, arms or other limbs to perform a repetitive task such as typing, clicking a mouse, texting or writing. The movements repeated day after day, year after year, thousand and thousands of times result in straining the muscles and tendons of the fingers or hands and microscopic tears are caused. The tendons become inflamed and begin to affect other nerves. As a result of this tingling, numbness can occur. If nothing is done about this cycle, repeated over and over, long term damage can occur.

"The Blackberry Thumb", as a result from too much typing on mobile devices is a frequently talked about topic amongst doctors and chiropractors. Now "text neck" is added to their vocabulary and is causing symptoms like neck strain, shoulder pain, headaches, and pain the arms and hands.

People hunch over their phone to text, play games, watch movies and they don't realise it could cause a debilitating pain for the rest of their lives. Fears are that the muscles are adapting to the flexed position so it becomes painful to have the neck in a normal position.

Chapter 2. Repetitive Strain Injury : An Overview

One of the main reasons why the hunching over or looking down on electronic devices can become painful is because of the weight of your head. A human head weighs 10 to 12 pounds or 4,5kg to 5,5kg. The neck and shoulders have to constantly take this weight and are not made to support that weight for hours and hours. Now this is especially a problem for children as their heads are larger than adults in relation to their body size.

RSIs can develop gradually over weeks, months, even years. Symptoms may come and go, making them difficult to pinpoint and even harder to diagnose. By the time they get to the doctor, people may be suffering from shooting pains, numb fingers, and muscle spasms. Due to the fact that their pain and limitations are invisible, people who suffer from RSIs may be seen as lazy and unwilling to do their share of the work.

For a long time, RSIs were found almost exclusively amongst workers who did physical work, especially cleaners, cooks, meatpackers, machine operators, and construction workers. When personal computers appeared on the desks of office workers in the 1980s, RSIs expanded into the office workforce. With the explosive popularity of computers for personal use, such as cell phones, PDAs, texting, game consoles, and other electronic devices, RSIs have spread into the general population. Research in Sweden found that one-half of the people who work with computers have pains in their necks, shoulders, arms, or hands.

There's another change in the population at risk: RSIs are no longer found only amongst adults. As young people participate more and more in the new technologies, growing numbers of children and teenagers are reporting aches, pains, and discomfort when using their computers, mobile phones, and video game consoles. An 8-year-old girl from Lancashire, UK, I who sends 30 text messages a day, for example, complained of pain in her fingers and wrists.

Attracted by the colours and images, even toddlers are drawn to computers. The long-term consequences for early computer users are not yet known, but medical experts fear that we may be raising generations of young adults who start their work lives already injured. What will happen as they age is the great unknown. Will they be able to work? Enjoy hobbies? Hold their children?

Chapter 2. Repetitive Strain Injury : An Overview

This is a BIG problem in this modern electronic society. Children sit down almost all day long as parents use the TV as their electronic baby sitter. As the small children grow older, they are given game consoles as an electronic baby sitter. Soon after that they will be receiving their first mobile phone followed by a laptop. No wonder RSI is a BIG problem these days and it will only become worse.

RSIs take a huge toll on individuals, affecting their jobs, financial stability, enjoyment of life, and personal relationships. The impaired functioning that can result in job loss also affects activities of daily living, such as carrying groceries, lifting a child, or dressing one's self. It is not uncommon for RSI sufferers to be unable to button their shirts or to tie their own shoes. Their social lives diminish as they become less and less able to participate in pleasurable activities. Depression, anger, frustration, and low self-esteem may accompany the pain and disability of RSIs. *As one 35-year-old woman lamented: "...RSI has destroyed my carefully built up confidence. I used to be a pretty happy person most of the time. I feel that I've permanently lost that person."*

RSI-sufferers story: *"...but my partner is desperately bored of my symptoms [sic] and finds me exceptionally annoying - and useless! He tells me to shut up 'cos he knows what I'm about to say - I'm a broken record. If he catches me having a whimper upstairs he rants and raves at me to grow up, change my job, get an operation. Although I would appreciate his sympathy occasionally I sort of understand where he's coming from - it must be tedious to have someone whining [sic]away doing the most mundane of chores!"* Source: Watson, M. 2009. Investigating the experiences of people with RSI. http://etheses.qmu.ac.uk/133/
RSIs are more common than most people think.

2. Statistics and facts
- Six people in the UK leave their jobs every day due to RSI. Source: Keytools

- Over half of adults in the U.S. reported a musculoskeletal condition in 2009. Source: Centres for Disease Control and Prevention.

- Ten percent of the sick notes written in London are for RSIs. Source: - London Evening Standard

Chapter 2. Repetitive Strain Injury : An Overview

- From 1996 to 2004, managing musculoskeletal diseases, including lost wages, cost an average $850 billion each year. Source: U.S. Department of Health.

- Office ergonomics training can reduce the average cost per workers' compensation claims by 90 percent, according to at least one study. Source: International Journal of Industrial Ergonomics Claims Management Company www.antriumlegal.com

- 30 percent of frequent computer users complain of tingling, burning or numbness of limbs. Source: American Family Physician

- 10 percent of frequent computer users have carpal tunnel syndrome, which is just one of many different types of RSIs. Source: American Family Physician

- In 2006, 450,000 workers in the UK (that's nearly one out of every 50 workers) reported RSIs. Source: Chartered Society of Physiotherapy

- British workers lost 3.5 million working days from RSIs in 2006-07 alone, at a cost of between £300 million. Source: Chartered Society of Physiotherapy

- Musculoskeletal disorders and diseases are the leading cause of disability in the United States and account for more than 50 percent of all chronic conditions in people over 50 years of age in developed countries. Source: American Academy of Orthopaedic Surgeons

- One out of every 50 workers in the UK have reported symptoms of RSIs. Source: Repetitive Strain Injury Association.

- 5.4 million working days are lost due to RSIs every year in the UK. Source: Repetitive Strain Injury Association.

- 45 percent of Irish workers have experienced RSI. Source: Siliconrepublic.com

www.repetitivestraininjuryhelp.com says:

- Globally, the most conventional approximation of related cost of repetitive strain injury disorders run into thousands of millions of dollars.

Chapter 2. Repetitive Strain Injury : An Overview

- Approximately, 63% of all office employees spend their most of time in holding mouse than any other device.

- More than 100 million individuals worldwide are predicted to suffer from some type of RSI or other computer associated health problems.

- According to recent surveys, insufficient breaks while working on system are the key factors responsible for encouraging the development of repetitive strain injury.

- RSI is unlikely to develop in single form, in several reports it has been established that the combination of lots of factors contribute to the repetitive strain injury risks.

- Taking regular breaks from working and releasing pressure on forearms, wrists and hands has seemed beneficial.

- The efficacy of most of preventative measures and ergonomics are disputed. No researches have presented these measures to be effectual in avoiding repetitive strain injury so far.

Cost involved in preventing RSI - according to www.repetitivestraininjuryhelp.com:

Now-a-days, huge money is being invested for avoiding the risk of RSI as governments and employees have been becoming aware about the widespread effects of this problem. Several RSI research studies suggest that ergonomic is one of the helpful ways to prevent RSI. They have also established that for every one dollar spent in RSI prevention, there is a return of approximately 17 dollars. **A** wide variety of ergonomics has been introduced ranging from armrests to keyboards costing about 100 dollars to other complete ergonomics desktops costing thousands of dollars.

It is really very difficult to figure out the exact amount that the government of a nation spends for preventing RSI. In the UK, almost 8 to 30 million USD are invested for treatment or preventing RSI while in the USA, this amount goes to 40 million USD. In European Union, about 40 to 60 millions USD are spend on RSI.

Chapter 2. Repetitive Strain Injury : An Overview

3. Anatomy of a Repetitive Strain Injury

Repetitive strain injuries affect the body's nerves and soft tissues—the muscles, ligaments and tendons. When repeated hundreds and thousands of times without ample time for recovery, simple movements damage the soft tissue. Muscles constrict from tiny tears and lubrication of tendons sheaths dry up. Inflamed tissues impinge on nerves, sending pain messages to the brain. Unlike an acute injury, repetitive strain injury develops gradually, without a definite starting point.

The human body has great powers to heal and restore itself, but when it does not have enough time to recover from small traumas and when the damaging conditions (that is, the risk factors) continue, the body cannot heal. That's what happens with RSIs.

The wrist and hand work via a complex system of tunnels and pulleys through which the tendons move to open and close the hand. For example, seven tendons pass through the carpal tunnel--from the wrist to the hand—to operate the fingers.

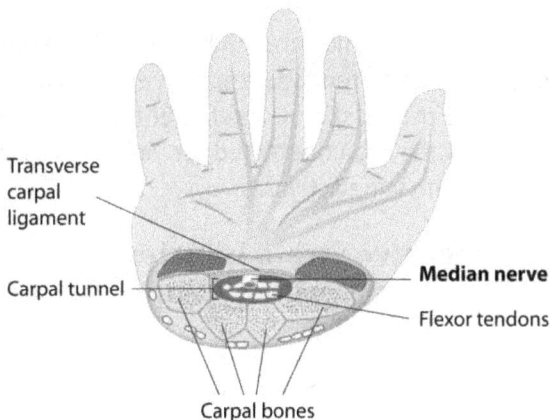

Tendons are strong and narrow rope-like cords that connect muscle and bone. They don't move very much; rather, they transfer movement from the muscles ("the powerhouse of the body") to the bones. A sheath that contains a lubricant called synovial fluid surrounds the tendons of the wrist and hand. The tendons move slightly within the sheath. With overuse the lubricant wears out, leaving the tendon rubbing against the sheath. The result is inflammation—hot, tender, and painful. As inflamed tissue expands it may also press on nerves, causing more pain along with numbness and tingling.

Ligaments are strong fibrous cords connecting bones to each other, forming joints. Ligaments reinforce and stabilise the joints. Working with the tendons, ligaments give motion to the joints of the wrist, elbow, and shoulder. When a joint moves beyond its normal range of motion, small tears occur in some of the ligament fibres. Damaged ligament fibres make the joint unstable, and take a long time to heal. Ligaments are protected by synovial fluid, but with repeated overuse friction between moving parts can cause inflammation.

Inflammation is one of the ways in which the body tries to heal itself. When tissues are damaged, extra blood flows in to repair the damage. Increased muscle tension and nerve constriction limit motion and cause pain. If it's not allowed to repair itself, that is, if overuse continues, scar tissue forms. Scar tissue shortens the forearms, putting stress on the tendons and because tendons are not very elastic, they rub on other tissue and become inflamed. Inflamed tissue swells and presses on nerves, damaging the nerves and causing pain.

Unlike sprains and strains, which are the result of single damaging events to the ligaments and tendons respectively, RSIs develop from small traumas (micro traumas) that occur over time. As each event is so small, the damage may go undetected for years, whilst individuals continue doing the damaging activities.

4. Types of Repetitive Strain Injuries
A number of different conditions that affect the soft tissues of the body fall under the RSI umbrella.

The most commonly occurring types of RSI are:

a) Carpal Tunnel Syndrome (CTS)
This is pressure on the median nerve as it passes through a passageway (the carpal tunnel, made up of ligament and bone) between the wrist and the hand. CTS usually starts with an ache in the wrist that may go up your hand or forearm. You may feel tingling or numbness in your thumb, fingers (except the little finger), or hand. Due to weakness in

the hand you may drop objects you try to pick up or hold. The tingling or numbness usually occurs when holding something or upon awakening. People may shake out their hands to try to relieve the symptoms. Over time the numbness may become constant. Pain may radiate from fingers to shoulder. Women are three times more likely to develop Carpal Tunnel Syndrome than men, possibly because the carpal tunnel is smaller in women. Doctors may prescribe wrist splints for CTS, which are usually worn at night to prevent the wrist from flexing during sleep. Tarsal tunnel syndrome is a similar nerve condition, but of the foot.

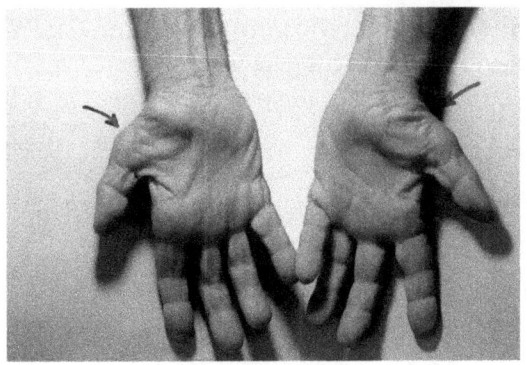

Untreated Carpal Tunnel Syndrome Source : http://upload.wikimedia.org/wikipedia/commons/thumb/6/68/Untreated_Carpal_Tunnel_Syndrome.JPG/1024px-Untreated_Carpal_Tunnel_Syndrome.JPG

b) Tendonitis (also, tendinitis)

This is inflammation of a tendon, which is the cord that connects muscle to bone. When tendons are overused or kept in one position for long periods of time, they can become inflamed or develop small tears. Tendonitis can occur anywhere that there is a tendon, but it is most common at the base of the thumb, elbow, shoulder, knee, hips, and Achilles tendon. The tendons of the hand and wrist are very small, putting them at high risk for repetitive strain injuries. Symptoms include a dull ache, tenderness, and mild swelling. Pain may increase gradually or it may be sudden and severe. People with tendonitis of their hands may not be able to hold onto objects. Individuals become more vulnerable to tendonitis as they age.

c) Tenosynovitis

Inflammation of the inner lining of the tendon sheath; most common in the hand, wrist, forearm or foot. With overuse, the tendons produce excess synovial fluid (which lines the tendon sheath), swelling the sheath and causing pain. Symptoms include joint pain, swelling, and/or stiffness; difficulty in moving a joint; pain and stiffness in the wrist on the thumb side; pain when moving a joint; and redness along the length of a tendon. The finger may stick in a bent position, a condition called "trigger finger." If tenosynovitis goes untreated, the tendon may tear, causing the joint to stiffen.

d) Diffuse RSI or non-specific pain syndrome (NSPS)

These are RSIs with no clear-cut diagnoses. People experience upper limb pain and dysfunction, but the pain is not focused in any one part of the body.

Less common RSIs include:

e) Bursitis

Inflammation and swelling of the fluid-filled sac (the bursa) near the joint of the knee, elbow, or shoulder.

f) Cubital Tunnel Syndrome

Loss of sensation, numbness, tingling, and muscle atrophy amongst people who work with elbows bent at 90 degrees for long periods of time. Sometimes confused with epicondylitis.

g) Epicondylitis

Inflammation of the area where bone and tendon meet on the inside or outside of the elbow, often caused by working with the elbows raised. Common among computer mouse users. Symptoms include severe pain when straightening arms. Golfer's elbow is a type of epicondylitis.

h) De Quervain's Syndrome

Excessive rubbing of the thumb tendons and their sheath causes pain over the thumb side of wrist, which may radiate up the arm. Also called DeQuervain's tenosynovitis.

i) Rotator Cuff Tendonitis

Chapter 2. Repetitive Strain Injury : An Overview

Inflammation of muscles and tendons of the shoulder, usually due to holding elbows away from the body for long periods of time.

j) Thoracic Outlet Syndrome
Numbness and tingling of the hand or hands due to compression of arteries and nerves, often made worse by reaching overhead.

5. Risk Factors
There is no single cause for RSIs, but there are factors that increase the risk for injury. Risk factors are events or conditions that increase the likelihood of a disorder occurring, but are not necessarily the cause. **Basically anybody who carries out the same movement over and over for years and years is at risk.** The risk factors for RSIs include:

a) Poorly designed workstations or tools.

b) Working for long periods of time without enough breaks.

c) Repetitive movements
- holding one's phone between neck and shoulder all day

- carrying heavy items

- texting all day long

- sitting in the same position for too long

- using a laptop for hours without breaks

- reading or using a laptop while looking down

- watching TV, in an incorrect position, without moving

- using a sewing machine whilst looking down for hours

- working on a PC for hours without a break

d) Awkward or constrained posture.

e) Fast work.

f) Staying in one position for too long.

g) Forceful exertions, including gripping.

Chapter 2. Repetitive Strain Injury : An Overview

h) Additional factors
Keep in mind that these RSI risk factors are not found just amongst workers and in computer users. Violinist Annie Mahtani had to give up a dynamic career at the age of 24 because of a repetitive strain injury in her wrist. She is not alone: At least 50 percent of orchestra musicians suffer from RSIs during their careers. Pianists are also very vulnerable to get RSI.

Swimmers, runners, and gymnasts are no strangers to RSIs. Racket sports can lead to tendonitis and tenosynovitis. You can get repetitive strain injury from knitting, gardening or playing guitar. Any activity, whether a job or hobby, that includes the risk factors listed above can lead to repetitive strain injury.

Personal factors can also contribute to an individual's risk for RSI. Certain diseases or conditions--such as rheumatoid arthritis, diabetes, thyroid disease, osteoporosis, and hyper-mobile joints--make it more likely that a person will develop RSI. Lack of physical fitness, pregnancy, and obesity also can contribute to RSIs, as can smoking and excessive use of alcohol. Medications that contribute to water retention, such as oral contraceptives, anti-inflammatory drugs, and blood pressure medication, can contribute to nerve compression, adding to the risk for RSIs.

Women are more vulnerable to RSIs than men, but that is most likely because women's muscles are usually smaller and therefore more easily damaged. People can get RSIs at any age; the rate of injury may be higher amongst older people simply because they have been participating in the damaging activity for a longer time. There may be a genetic component to RSIs but studies are still ongoing.

Stress, both physical and psychosocial, increase the risk for injury. Relationships on the job, conflict at work, work demands that exceed the workers' abilities, financial insecurity, problems at home, and job dissatisfaction can contribute to the development of RSIs.

6. Symptoms of RSI
RSIs are progressive: they get worse over time and they rarely get better on their own. They can, however, be treated. If you recognise the repetitive strain injury symptoms early, you can get treatment

Chapter 2. Repetitive Strain Injury : An Overview

before you become disabled. The sooner you start treatment, the more successful the treatment is likely to be.

When you first notice symptoms of RSI, unfortunately you have already done substantial damage to your body.

Symptoms of the different types of RSIs differ, but there are a number of typical early RSI indicators. Many RSI suffers find that symptoms come and go seemingly without explanation because RSIs develop gradually, often over a long period of time, the early symptoms are often overlooked.

a) Early signs

- **Aches, pains, cramps, swelling or tenderness in muscles or joints.** Pain may be mild or severe; it may be burning or shooting. You may feel pain in specific locations, like your fingers or you may feel it along your entire arm and hand. Pain may move and be hard to pinpoint. You may have pain in areas of the body distant from the site of the injury e.g. you may get a pain in your upper neck but the real problem is in the muscle of your lower neck.

- **Fatigue.** RSI sufferers may get tired from activities they could previously do for long periods of time without difficulty.

- **Headaches.** If you get the headaches only when you are doing your repetitive movements, it could be a sign that some muscles in your neck are not working properly. Headaches on top of your head or on one side of your head (left or right forehead) are often a sign of damage to certain muscles. Trigger point massage or deep tissue can be very helpful for this.

- **Weakness of the arms.** Weakness can make it hard to do simple tasks. When weakness affects grip strength, sufferers may need two hands to hold onto objects.

- **Restricted movement of limbs.** Difficulty opening and closing your hands or using your hands for normal activities can be a sign of an RSI.

- **Cold hands.** Cold hands can indicate nerve damage.

Chapter 2. Repetitive Strain Injury : An Overview

- **Hypersensitivity.** A light touch over a strained muscle or tendon may feel painful.

- **Reduced sensation.** On the other end of the spectrum from hypersensitivity is diminished feeling in the fingers.

b) Later symptoms

- **Numbness and/or tingling.** When hands often feel like they have fallen asleep it may be a sign of nerve damage.

- **Spasms, tremors, and/or twitching in the forearms.**

- **Continuous pain in the affected area, even without movement.** The pain may be severe enough to wake the RSI sufferer up during the night.

> **The worst thing is I can't even pick up my new born baby.**

- **Difficulty holding onto objects.** When the arms and hands become weaker, RSI sufferers may find themselves dropping simple objects like coffee cups or pens. They may not have the strength to pick up a sack of groceries or even hold onto a child.

c) Continuum of Symptoms

In their book Repetitive Strain Injury: A Computer User's Guide, Dr. Emil Pascarelli and Deborah Quilter outline a continuum of RSI that describes the symptoms and the typical course of untreated RSIs.

- Pre-RSI: "Funny" feeling in arms or hands, relieved by rest.

- Early RSI: Intermittent pain or tingling while typing, relieved by rest and rehabilitation.

- Danger Zone: Weakness, clumsiness, intermittent pain not necessarily relieved by rest; daily activities impaired; depression. Moderate risk of permanent impairment.

- Chronic Pain: Weakness, constant pain, not relieved by rest and made worse by any activity. High risk of permanent impairment and disability.

Chapter 2. Repetitive Strain Injury : An Overview

- Chronic Pain and Dysfunction: Chronic pain; depression, dystonia (painful involuntary contractions of the muscles); severe chronic pain with weakness, tremors, and spasms. Permanent disability.

d) Changes in Habits
RSI sufferers may change their habits or make excuses for their symptoms without even knowing it. They may start using paper plates so they don't risk dropping dishes. Or, they may change sports, like taking up jogging instead of playing tennis as they used to. They may say they can't pick up the baby because their back hurts. They may stop wearing neckties, saying they prefer the casual look when in reality it's because they can no longer knot their ties. People who suffer from RSIs may not realize that they are changing their lives to accommodate their injuries but it should be changing their lives to prevent them.

RSI-sufferer's story: "I was rinsing off some spaghetti the other night and my fingers in the affected hand just let go of the colander - and the spaghetti landed in the sink. That was the end of another meal! I can't cut up my food properly or clean my teeth very well (although I have now bought a sonic wave toothbrush which helps with this task). When the pain and motor function is really bad, it's embarrassing to have to ask someone to unzip/unbutton my jeans or trousers so I can go to the loo, or having to ask my husband to cut up my food for me because I can't manage to do this simple task myself." Source: Watson, M. 2009. Investigating the experiences of people with RSI. http://etheses.qmu.ac.uk/

7. RSI and Arthritis
The relationship between RSIs and arthritis is complex, with more research needed to completely understand the connections.

Here are some of the current research findings about RSIs and arthritis:

- Major risk factors for RSIs—namely, overuse and repetitive motion—are also risk factors for osteoarthritis, the most common type of arthritis. Activities like keying that involve repeating the same movements for long periods of time not only lead to RSIs, but can also lead to arthritis in the hands, shoulders, fingers, elbows and wrists.

Chapter 2. Repetitive Strain Injury : An Overview

Sitting at a desk for long periods of time can also contribute to both arthritis and RSIs.

- Like RSIs, osteoarthritis involves the gradual accumulation of minor daily wear and tear. In fact, osteoarthritis is also called wear-and-tear arthritis, alluding to the overuse factor.

- Carpal tunnel syndrome is a common problem for people with rheumatoid arthritis, a chronic inflammatory condition. Inflammation of the tendons of the wrist compresses the nerve, leading to weakness, loss of dexterity and pain and numbness during the night. Source: Techniques in Orthopaedics: March 2006 - Volume 21 - Issue 1 - pp 42-47doi: 10.1097/01.bto.0000220073.29489.6c

- Rheumatoid arthritis is the most common non-occupational risk factor for carpal tunnel syndrome.

- Some of the symptoms of RSIs and arthritis are the same, especially pain in the thumbs and other joints. Arthritic conditions, including rheumatoid arthritis and osteoarthritis, can all cause pain in the hands and fingers that may look like carpal tunnel syndrome. The treatments for the different conditions are however, not the same. Source: Carpal Tunnel SyndromeNYTimesshttp://health.nytimes.com/health/guides/disease/carpal-tunnel-syndrome/diagnosis.htm

- Osteoarthritis is one of several diseases that increase the risk for RSIs. Repetitive strain injury is more likely in someone with osteoarthritis. A recent study found an elevated risk for RSIs among workers with arthritis. Source: Journal of Occupational & Environmental Medicine: July 2012 - Volume 54 - Issue 7 - p 841–846 doi: 10.1097/JOM.0b013e31824e11f

Just with RSIs, ergonomic design of workstations can make it easier for people with arthritis to do their jobs. Discussing ergonomic design for workers with arthritis, Dr. Diane Lacaille at the Arthritis Research Centre of Canada found that "workers whose workspaces had been ergonomically modified to be more comfortable were 60 percent less likely to be away from work due to disability." Source: The Arthritis Society. Researcher aims to prevent arthritis-related work disability.

Chapter 2. Repetitive Strain Injury : An Overview

http://www.arthritis.ca/look%20at%20research/researcherssummary/dianelacaille/default.asp?s=1&province=sk)

RSI-sufferers story: "After years of typing, it came out of nowhere: an aching, stabbing, tingling pain in my arms and hands. My primary complaint was a throbbing ache followed by pinpricks of fiery pain on my fingers, like someone putting out cigarettes on my skin. I couldn't work with my hands in any capacity, and I couldn't sleep. Nothing seemed to work to alleviate the pain. Not ibuprofen, not acetaminophen, not painkillers. I had carpal tunnel.

"...I underwent surgery, therapy, and ergonomic mindfulness. Once I started typing again at full force, though, it all started coming back. As it stands, I've got the odds stacked against me: I'm a woman, a writer, a guitarist, and I have a genetic predisposition to carpal tunnel, tendonitis, and arthritis. A perfect storm for pain.

"It was a second doctor who suggested vitamin B6, which, I'm happy to report, makes daily life tolerable...However, there are still some things I can no longer do (playing guitar, folding laundry, using a regular keyboard, reading heavy books, picking up my son, prolonged vegetable chopping). I get by, though not without some major readjusting. I've had to restructure my writing process, the way I play music, and even how I interact with my kids. I can't tell you how heartbreaking it is to walk into a guitar store these days. After playing for eighteen years, I've had to give it up entirely or else spend three days in pain after jamming. It's just not worth it." Source: Natania Barron at wired.com 26 July 2012.

Chapter 3. Treatment of RSIs

1. Treatment Issues

Many people ignore the early signs of RSIs ; the dull aches and pains that go away with rest. However, the sooner you recognize the symptoms, the easier it is to treat the problem. If you stop doing the activity that is causing the stress and discomfort, you may be able to relieve the symptoms with self-care. Once the RSI progresses you will most likely need medical attention. Treating later stages (when there is numbness, tingling, and continuous pain) is more difficult and often less successful than treating RSIs in the early stages.

Recovery from RSI is a very slow process; it takes time to repair the damage to the body. In addition recovery is not a straight line; it's often two steps forward and one step back, as one man with RSI describes: "...it keeps me on the emotional rollercoaster that life has become[.] just when I think I'm getting better, or coming out of an episode I have a bad day and I can't explain it." Source: Watson, M. 2009. Investigating the experiences of people with RSI. http://etheses.qmu.ac.uk/133/

Too often people with RSIs get encouraged by small improvements and overdo it, delaying recovery even more. For any treatment to work, it is necessary to stop or change the behaviour that led to the injury. That's just the beginning of the long and slow path to recovery.

There's more to be learned about the treatment of RSIs. Clinical trials are underway in a number of countries, including the United Kingdom and the United States. You can find out about clinical trials through the NHS at http://www.nhs.uk/conditions/repetitive-strain-injury/Pages/Introduction.aspx.

RSI-sufferers have found relief, even cure, from a variety of treatment modalities. What works for one person may not work for another, so you may have to try out different treatments before you find one (or a combination) that works for you. Wrong diagnosis and inappropriate treatment can make RSIs worse, so individuals should consult a medical professional before undergoing any type of treatment. This is important to rule out any other health issue.

Chapter 3. Treatment of RSIs

2. Choosing a Doctor

Not all medical providers understand RSIs, so it may be wise to get more than one professional opinion or seek out a provider with a reputation for the successful treatment of RSIs. A good relationship with your medical provider is essential to RSI treatment. That's because there's no single way to treat a repetitive strain injury; it may take some trial and error, and for that you need to have open communication with your doctor. You'll want someone who is a good listener, is sympathetic, and has time to spend with you.

It is perfectly acceptable to ask questions about a doctor before, to help you decide if you want to work with him or her. You may ask questions such as:

- What is your experience in treating repetitive strain injuries?

- What treatments do you find most effective?

- How can I contact you between visits if I need help or information?

- Are you willing to work with my insurance company and/or employer?

- What specialists do you work with on RSIs?

Many people find it helpful to bring someone with them when they go to a doctor, particularly when they are seeing a new doctor or discussing treatment options. It's very difficult to take in everything a doctor tells you, especially when you're upset; a second set of ears can help you. The person you bring with you should be sympathetic to your situation, a good listener, and able to ask relevant questions without interfering. He or she should have a reasonable understanding of your condition. You may want to ask this person to take notes, or you may want to bring a voice recorder with you to your appointments.

Your doctor may refer you to specialists such as a neurologist, rheumatologist, occupational physician, sports medicine doctor, or physiatrist. (Physiatrists treat conditions that affect how you move, providing non-surgical therapies and pain management.) Your doctor may suggest seeing a mental health care provider for help with

Chapter 3. Treatment of RSIs

depression or to help you develop tools for coping with your RSI. He or she may refer you for occupational or physical therapy, deep tissue massage, or any number of the treatment options listed below. You want to be sure that the doctor you choose to work with will communicate with all the specialists and providers and coordinate your care.

You and your doctor must work as a team to make sure that you get the services you need for your recovery. You can do your part by keeping a journal of your symptoms and treatments, what makes symptoms worse and what makes them better; by keeping a list of medications; and by educating yourself about your RSI and options for effective treatment. Websites for More Information about RSIs, at the end of this book, are a good starting place for learning more about he condition. Keep records of all your medical visits, medications, and tests and test results. Being an active participant in your recovery is part of the healing process.

RSI-sufferer's story: *"I eventually persuaded my GP to refer me to a rheumatologist. I felt saved at this point because I was sure I must have something like this wrong with me. I was actually disappointed when the results [from the GP] came back negative as I so wanted somebody to tell me that I wasn't mad and that there was something wrong with me."* Source: Watson, M. 2009. Investigating the experiences of people with RSI. http://etheses.qmu.ac.uk/133/

RSI-sufferers story: "Doctors have disagreed with each other, and blamed each other for not doing the right thing. My employers don't know what to believe. I feel like my employers have written me off. My doctor told me to hang my job up. That's a huge decision." Source: Repetitive Strain Injury: A Computer User's Guide by Emil Pascarelli, MD and Deborah Quilter.

3. Conventional Treatments

Diagnosis by a medical professional should guide treatment. Diagnosis explains the symptoms and opens up different treatment options. The effectiveness of the different treatments varies with the individual and with the type of RSI. The most common treatment options are as follows:

Chapter 3. Treatment of RSIs

a) Physiotherapy
Light, infrared and ultraviolet rays, heat, electric current, massage, manipulation, and exercise.

b) Extended Scope Physiotherapy (ESP)
ESP practitioners study beyond the requirements of regular physiotherapists. They can request investigations such as nerve conduction scans and assist in diagnosis and treatment, listing for surgery, and referrals to other medical professionals.

c) Medication
Muscle relaxants and nonsteroidal anti-inflammatory drugs (NSAIDs) such as naproxen and ibuprofen reduce pain and swelling.

d) Immobilization
Lessens pain by immobilizing hands and arms with wrist braces, splints or elastic wrist supports. Often used at night with carpal tunnel syndrome. If overused, splints et al can do more damage than good, so should only be used on medical order.

e) Hypnosis
Pain management and healing in which patients visualize images that promote healing.

f) Heat packs
Heat packs can relieve chronic pain and relax muscles. May be used in combination with cold packs.

g) Steroid injections
Corticosteroid is injected into soft tissue for short-term pain relief. Steroid injections can have negative side effects and should be considered carefully.

h) Chiropractic and osteopathic manipulation
Manipulate joints and muscles to restore them to normal positions and relieve tension.

i) Deep tissue massage
Relieves severe tension in the muscle connective tissue (called the fascia), focusing on the tissue below the surface muscles.

j) Trigger point massage/therapy

Chapter 3. Treatment of RSIs

Releases painful trigger points (or muscle knots) that are the source of referred pain. Trigger points are tiny points in the muscle that are tender when touched.

k) Ultrasound therapy
High-intensity ultrasound can reduce pain and improve the healing of carpal tunnel syndrome and tendonitis. Ultrasound can also be used to aid the placement of cortisone injections.

l) Physical therapy
Stretching and strengthening exercises to reduce stress and recondition the body. This may also include postural retraining, ultrasound, heat and ice packs, or deep tissue massage.

m) Occupational therapy
Exercises and training focused on helping people with activities of daily living.

n) Tiger Balm
Tiger Balm is wrapped on the painful areas and can give temporary relief.

o) Firm Splints
A splint is a device used for support or immobilization of the spine or other limbs.

p) Surgery
Carpal Tunnel Syndrome surgery may be recommended if symptoms last for a period of six months or longer. Physicians may also recommend RSI surgery for other advanced conditions. Surgery for RSIs are not always effective (the failure rate is over 50 percent) and is usually considered as a last resort.

Chapter 3. Treatment of RSIs

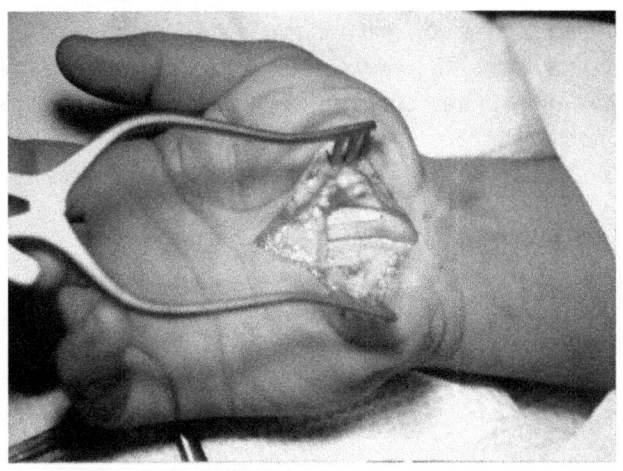

Carpal Tunnel Surgery Source:
http://commons.wikimedia.org/wiki/File:Carpal_Tunnel_Syndrome,_Operatio
n.jpg

4. Complementary/Alternative Treatments

Complementary and alternative therapies help people with RSI to recover from symptoms and deal with their injuries on a daily basis. The line between traditional and conventional/alternative treatments is not always well defined. Individuals should discuss such treatments with their physician.

Such treatments, which are often used in conjunction with conventional treatments, include:

a) Alexander technique

Postural retraining increases awareness of body position, making it easier to assume safe positions for computer use.

Sufferer's story: *With hindsight, I think I was fast heading for Chronic Fatigue Syndrome, and I don't know how I was coping with that degree of chronic exhaustion: in short, not well. Constantly uncomfortable. Sleep disturbance most nights. Uncharacteristically feeling awful in the mornings. Depression (small d): feeling dull, with a very narrow emotional range, usually feeling very little of anything except discomfort, pain and irritation and frustration with those around me. Beginning to feel a bit dependent and helpless. Very low energy levels. Emotionally drained. (I could hardly smile.) Finding it progressively* more difficult to do creative work as a writer of fiction. **Numbness and pain in hands, arms, shoulders, neck, back. Numb feet and burning sensations in my knees.** Clenched neck and shoulders, unable to let go. Chronic tensions throughout my body, from feet and crackling ankles upwards. Clicks and cracks and crunches, and sometimes intolerable pressure in my pelvic area. Unable to sit still for more than two minutes.

Dinner parties, where I had to sit still for hours, were torture, and I found myself unable to focus on the conversation at all, and felt desperate for everyone to go home and leave me alone. I bumped into things regularly, and fumbled often. I could hardly get change out of my wallet-- that kind of manual dexterity simply wasn't available. After struggling to do so, my lower back and collar bone area would be numb and profoundly uncomfortable. Brushing my teeth was so daunting that I frequently didn't. I couldn't do anything, not even exercise, without discomfort.

Doors of opportunity seemed to be slamming shut on me almost daily, and my options for a career seemed to be dwindling almost to nothing.

I was in need of company in order to feel okay, but I must have been terrible to have around. My friends were patient, but uncomprehending and embarrassed, not knowing what to say, or how to respond to the answer. The subject was mostly just dropped as compassion fatigue set in and I was left to cope with it on my own.

I got a lot of pain relief from The Alexander technique. Source: www.alexandertechnique.com

b) Biofeedback
Measures stresses and offers methods for relaxing mind and muscles.

c) Cognitive Behavioural Therapy (CBT)
Approach to controlling and managing pain and depression.

d) Pilates
Body conditioning targets deep abdominal muscles to build strength and improve flexibility.

e) Yoga

Chapter 3. Treatment of RSIs

Helps with fitness, strengthening, and flexibility. Reduces pain and improves grip strength for people with carpal tunnel syndrome.

f) Tai Chi
Improves posture with moving meditation/martial art. It strengthens muscles, improves flexibility, and stimulates healing.

g) Bowen Technique
Promotes rebalancing and proper alignment. RSI-sufferers who find most touch painful may like the very gentle touch of the Bowen Technique.

h) Feldenkrais Method
Improves body awareness through bodywork and gentle exercise. Retrains the body, making all movements smooth and efficient.

i) Shiatsu
Japanese finger pressure therapy targets acupuncture points.

j) Acupuncture
Removes energy blockages, relieves aches and pains, and promotes relaxation and general well being.

k) Reflexology
Removes blockages in nerve endings, allowing nerves to function better.

l) Craniosacral Therapy
Removes restrictions in cerebrospinal fluid and energy flow in the body.

m) Magnet Therapy
Increases circulation, which helps the healing process.

n) Relaxation Techniques
Reduce physical and mental stress, tension, and pain.

An RSI-sufferer's story: *My name is Judith Kay. I'm a professional singer/guitarist and composer of jazz-style music...I have been dealing with repetitive strain injury for the better part of 20 years...When I was first hit hard with this condition in 1992, I was totally confused by what was happening to me. I just knew that, suddenly, to do almost anything* *with my hands put me in excruciating pain. Almost in a daze, I went from doctor to therapist to doctor, getting little or no help and sometimes very bad recommendations about what to do...I had electric shock type pain up my arm when just touching something lightly, or would feel an eerily strange buzzing sensation. My pain level escalated often to a horrifying level 9 or 10, and stayed there. I could not open a drawer or a door, and I could barely comb my hair or brush my own teeth, and was certainly unable to prepare my own food.*

In just two months time of regular visits [for deep tissue massage] my pain level was significantly decreased and I was well on the road to recovery... A few months after that I was back to driving and performing most activities of daily living without pain. A short time after that I began playing the guitar again. Of course there was an important daily regimen of exercises that got me to this place.." source:http://www.judithkay.com/repetitivestraininjury.htm.

o) Understanding Pain Syndromes
The Mind Body Prescription is a book by Dr. John E. Sarno about pain syndromes such as RSI. Some people say if they understand the pain they can deal with it better.

p) Walking or moving
Listed last but certainly not the least important: you will be surprised how much good walking can do for your body. Get yourself to a park or just go for a walk outside your house.

5. Self Care
No matter what types of treatments you pursue, you will need to add a big dose of self-care to your RSI recovery programme. Doctors and therapists will provide information, support, therapies and assistance, but you will have to follow through. Recovery from RSI requires life changes, which **ONLY YOU** can make.

To give your body the best chance of recovery, pay attention to your overall health and wellbeing. If you feel pain or discomfort whilst performing a certain task or activity, stop immediately and take a break. Be sure to give the affected area plenty of rest. Avoid activities that make symptoms worse. Many RSI-sufferers report feeling so much

Chapter 3. Treatment of RSIs

better after taking a walk, no matter how long or how vigorous the walk is.

Most important of all, be kind to yourself. An RSI does not make you a bad or lazy person. You are the same person you were before you became injured. Have sympathy for yourself, but don't wallow in self-pity. It's a challenging but important balance: have empathy for your situation but don't feel like a victim.

Analyse if you can do things differently e.g.

- instead of sending an email, use the phone

- instead of sending a message, get out of your chair and go and speak to the person.

- Stop playing solitaire on your laptop or PC and get yourself an old fashioned set of playing cards, much more fun and much more sociable!

- Stop chatting on Facebook and arrange to meet up somewhere so you can do the chatting whilst socialising.

- Stop surfing the web and get information the old fashioned way: from the library, magazines or from books.

To summarise: try and eliminate the time you spend using your laptop or mobile phone.

The most important thing is to realise what exactly gives you pain and reduce the time you are doing that activity. Stop the motions that caused the injury in the first place.

Chapter 3. Treatment of RSIs

You absolutely MUST take plenty of breaks doing the same thing.

You absolutely MUST do some gentle exercises rather than sitting on your bed or in front of your laptop all day long.

You absolutely must sit in the correct posture when using a laptop or a PC.

Chapter 4. Coping with a Repetitive Strain Injury

RSI-sufferers story: *"I don't actually know how I coped - I just did. My husband had to do many extra chores - I couldn't chop vegetables, I would drop things and break many jars/plates/glasses in the kitchen, turning keys in locks was impossible with my right hand - as was general things like doing up bra straps, washing and drying my hair. I think I coped because I had to look after this baby..."* Source: Watson, M. 2009. Investigating the experiences of people with RSI. http://etheses.qmu.ac.uk/133/

Simple coping strategies can make life so much easier. The overall coping strategy is to be aware of what works for you and what doesn't, take breaks before you hurt, and use your body gently.

For additional practical tips, go to JAN (the Job Accommodation Network); this website has a searchable database of ideas and accommodations, at https://askjan.org/media/cumu.htm. The Vendors list at the end of this book includes companies that sell devices for daily living.

Insurance, work benefits, and/or other benefit programs may cover the cost of some of the products and services you need to cope with your disability.

This chapter contains ideas from the experts: people who suffer from RSIs, arthritis and other conditions that limit the use of their arms and hands. You will have to experiment to find what works best for you—what's easiest, but checking out the tips below is a good place to start.

1. Shopping
- Buy groceries and supplies in smaller quantities so you don't have to do as much lifting and carrying.

- Make more trips instead of carrying too many bags at once.

- Shop at stores that deliver.

Chapter 4. Coping with a Repetitive Strain Injury

- Avoid shoulder bags for carrying. Use rucksacks that have two straps and a waistband for distributing your weight. Or use wheeled carry bags.

- Wear clothes with big pockets for carrying a few items.

- If you have to carry a bag, try resting the handle over your forearm instead of gripping the handle with your fingers. The muscles in the arm are bigger and stronger than those in your fingers, so they can do more work without injury.

2. Out in the World

- Shaking hands poses a dilemma for RSI-sufferers. A handshake can be painful for sore hands, but if the other person is a business associate or new acquaintance, you may not want them to know you can't shake hands and you don't want to seem rude. Here are ideas to solve the problem: you can gently put your hands around the other person's forearm, bow slightly, or hold a light object in your hand so it's obvious you can't shake. Your objective is to protect your hand without appearing discourteous.

- Instead of clapping, shout "bravo!" Or, stamp your feet, tap your palm with a program, or pretend to clap without actually touching your hands together. Or, try the applause used by deaf audiences: raise your hands, stretch out your fingers, and twist your wrists.

- If you take public transportation, avoid rush hour if you can so you can be sure of getting a seat. If you don't get a seat, put your bag between your feet instead of holding it; loop your arm around a pole instead of trying to hold on with your hands.

- Driving—don't do it unless you have complete control over your vehicle. Power steering; automatic transmission; and power windows, mirrors, locks, and seats make it easier.

- Use an easy reach seat belt handle to reach your seat belt without straining.

- Use feet and legs instead of hands to open and close doors. Push doors open with your hip, foot, or shoulder. As much as possible let other people open doors for you.

Chapter 4. Coping with a Repetitive Strain Injury

- Push doorbells and elevator buttons with an elbow, knuckle, or umbrella.

3. Communicating

- It's easy to become isolated by the pain and limitations of RSIs, so it's important to keep lines of communication open. Your familiar ways of communicating may become uncomfortable. Here are ideas for keeping in touch.

- Call people on the phone instead of sending emails or texts.

- Use handsets and speakerphones when talking on the telephone.

- Easy-touch keyboards take less hand effort.

- Use the auto-dial feature on the telephone, or get a voice-activated phone.

- Check with your telephone service provider. The disabilities services of phone companies in some locales may offer discounts to people with RSIs.

- For writing, choose pens that have thick, soft grips and write with very little pressure, like old-fashioned fountain pens. If you can't find thick enough pens wrap bubble wrap or a foam hair curler around a pen.

- Use a slop board angled at 10 degrees to minimise neck strain while you write.

- STOP TEXTING AND START TALKING.

The following ideas are adapted from hints from members of Australia's RSI Association:

Activity	Old Way	Alternative Ways
Letters and card writing	Pen and paper	Audiotape, pre-stamped envelopes, self-inking stamp or address labels, computer generated address labels.
Taking notes	Pen and paper	Audiotape, writing with other hand,

Chapter 4. Coping with a Repetitive Strain Injury

	Word processor	dictation
Journal/diary	Pen and paper Word processor	Talk to others to clarify thoughts and problems instead of writing them down. Use mind maps, drawings, etc. to portray your feelings. Audiotape.
Bill paying and banking	Pen and paper	Telephone banking, direct debit, direct deposit, online banking.

4. Dressing and Grooming

- Buy clothing with zippers instead of buttons and shoes that slip on or have Velcro closures instead of laces.

- Buy skirts and slacks with elastic waists.

- Avoid clothing that needs to be ironed. You can reduce wrinkles by hanging up clothes after you wear them or wash them, putting clothes in the dryer, or hanging them near the shower so steam can release wrinkles.

- Use a shoehorn. A shoe and boot valet lets you put on and take off shoes with one hand without bending down.

- Use a reaching tool to access, for example, socks on the floor or jumpers on high shelves.

- Store clothes on shelves instead of in bureau drawers.

- Zipper pulls, long handle hairbrushes, button pulls, and bra aids make grooming and dressing easier.

- Use one-handed nail clippers to keep nails trim; long fingernails interfere with good typing technique.

- Hang your head down when brushing or blow drying so you

Chapter 4. Coping with a Repetitive Strain Injury

don't have to raise your arms up.

- Repair hems, seams, and tears with fabric glue instead of needle and thread.

5. Around the House

- Use kitchen equipment with thicker, easier to grip handles. Wrap foam hair curlers, bubble wrap, or foam handles around pencils, pens, and eating utensils to make them easier to hold onto. OXO Good Grips (www.oxo.com) is a line of kitchen tools and dining utensils with soft, thick grips.

- Use bendable dining utensils for easier holding and cutting.

- Use double-handed mugs, which are easier to lift and hold on to.

- Use a bookstand so you don't have to hold the book in your hands.

- Use very sharp, serrated knives for dining and preparing food. They take less effort.

- Fit lamp switch enlargers over existing light switches to make them easier to grasp and turn.

- Use automatic staplers and spring-loaded scissors.

- Go electrical: can opener, knife sharpener, knives, card shuffler, razor, etc.

- Cover keys with key holders to make them easier to grip.

- Store frequently used items on shelves at waist level so you don't have to reach overhead for them. Items you use daily should stay on the countertop.

- Install door handle grips, turners, or extenders over round doorknobs. Turn the doorknob with finger, elbow, or closed fist. Available from Good Grips (http://www.greatgrips.com),

Chapter 4. Coping with a Repetitive Strain Injury

Assistive Devices Key (http://www.assistivedeviceskey.com/) and Life with Ease http://www.lifewithease.com/

6. Gardening

Gardening has both physical and psychological benefits: it gets your body moving and soothes your mind. You may have to adopt new gardening methods and tools; fortunately adaptive gardening has many practical tips and new and accomplished gardeners.

- Build raised bed gardens so you don't have to bend or reach so far. Thus, if you have mobility limitations you can still garden.

- Reduce the size of your garden. Compact gardens can be amazingly beautiful...and less work.

- Use a heavy mulch to reduce the amount of weeding, watering, and fertilizing you have to do.

- Instead of digging or roto-tilling your vegetable garden use the no-till method.

- Don't use power tools.

- Lightweight hand tools, long-handled tools, and padded handles all make tools easier to use.

- Pistol grips on hand tools and bent handles on digging tools help keep your hand in the neutral position and so need less force to use.

- Install a watering system so you don't have to carry a hose or watering can. Better still grow plants that thrive in your location without much water. If you do turn on a hose now and then install plastic fittings (tap turners) that make it easier.

- Avoid pruning by planting trees and shrubs that grow slowly and/or don't require annual trimming.

- Use wheelbarrows or garden carts for carrying. Don't overload them. It's better to make more trips than to strain your arms, hands, and shoulders with heavy loads.

Chapter 4. Coping with a Repetitive Strain Injury

- Never work to the point of pain. Pace yourself and take frequent breaks.

The American Horticultural Therapy Association (www.ahta.org), the Canadian Horticultural Therapy Association (www.chta.ca), and Trellis (www.trellisscotland.org.uk) focus on gardening for people with disabilities. As the American Horticultural Therapy Association website puts it: "The therapeutic benefits of peaceful garden environments have been understood since ancient times."

7. Managing Pain

RSIs are painful. The pain itself can be debilitating but most RSI-

> **My hands hurt so much I could cry.**

sufferers learn to manage the pain. Pain management is partly physical and partly mental and a number of the treatment options listed here are self-care techniques that you can use to deal with your pain.

- If it hurts when you do a certain activity, stop doing it but don't stop moving altogether. Moving keeps the blood circulating and speeds up recovery.

- Cold is a quick and easy way to temporarily reduce inflammation and swelling, and therefore pain. Use it straight after you do something that causes pain and for up to 15 times a day. Apply ice or cold water directly on the painful spot, but keep the ice moving (don't let it sit on your skin) for about a minute. Let the spot where you applied the ice warm up before you start an activity. Important note: cold treatment is only recommended when inflammation occurs. Heat is better for general aches and pains when there is no inflammation.

- Heat relaxes sore muscles and makes them easier to move. Use heat packs, warm water or hot water bottles for moist heat. You can buy microwavable heat packs, which a lot of people recommend.

- Some RSI-sufferers find temporary relief from TENS (Transcutaneous Electrical Nerve Stimulation) **machines. These**

Chapter 4. Coping with a Repetitive Strain Injury

machines send electrical impulses to parts of the body to block pain. They should only be used under the direction of a medical professional.

- Exercise relieves pain, speeds up healing, reduces stress, and decreases anxiety and depression. Try walking, swimming, yoga, or biking.

- Many people find listening to music soothing.

- Stretches and strengthening exercises relieve stress.

- Self-massage relieves pain. You can massage one hand/arm with the other hand, roll a hard rubber ball (tennis or squash ball) between your arm and a table or between your back and the floor, use a massage machine, or use simple massage tools.

- Professional massage relaxes muscles and reduces pain. The choice of massage is individual but many RSI sufferers prefer a light touch, although my mum simply loves deep tissue massage and always gets a lot of pain relief from it.

- Herbal oils, menthol creams, and rubbing ointments can soothe sore muscles and bring relief.

- Mind-body approaches to pain management use the power of thoughts and feelings to reduce pain and support healing. Biofeedback, meditation, and cognitive behaviour therapy (CBT) are three of many mind-body techniques that you can learn and practice on your own.

- Pain clinics can help with a variety of pain management techniques.

RSI-sufferers story: "By the fourth morning that I drag myself out of bed long before dawn, my self-pity has turned into actual concern. There's a screaming pain running across the back of my shoulders." Source: Mother Jones magazine, March/April 2012.

RSI-sufferers story: "By the end of the day, your body hurts so bad...You tell them you can't do it the next day, ... they'll tell you, 'We've got four more people waiting for your job.'...My

Chapter 4. Coping with a Repetitive Strain Injury

body still is not the same, I still have aches and I still have pains. I have migraines because of the stress I went through working at that place." Source: Huffington Post, 20 December 2011

8. Relaxation
Relaxation techniques and visualizations help individuals to relax in a deep way, which reduces stress, anxiety and pain. Conscious breathing is a simple and effective relaxation technique: Breathe into the tension in your body, then let the tension go as you breathe out. Imagine your shoulders, arms, and hands relaxing. A number of the alternative treatments listed above include relaxation techniques that you can learn and do by yourself.

You might try sitting or lying down in a quiet place and concentrating on feeling the pulse in one part of your body. Focus on relaxing and increasing the circulation to that spot. As you relax you may feel more pulse and more blood flow. Then move your attention to another part of your body.

9. Stretching and Exercising
Moving the body releases endorphins, which reduce pain. It also decreases tension and improves muscle strength. It gets blood flowing throughout the body, nourishing the tissues and aiding healing. Exercise improves overall wellbeing, relieves depression and makes the body less vulnerable to injury.

There are two parts to exercise: stretching and strengthening. The stretching exercises in different sections of this book are designed to relieve tension in the parts of the body you overuse when you text, type, or use other electronic devices. It only takes seconds to stretch, so you can do it many times a day. Stretch while you wait for the bus, in between phone calls, when you take breaks from computing, while a clerk rings you up—whenever you have a free moment. Stretching should start slow and easy, increasing with steady pressure and stopping just before the point of pain. No bouncing, jerking or quick movements. The simple stretches described in this book should not hurt; stop if they do and seek medical attention. If you have an RSI, your doctor may discourage certain stretches, especially if you are in the acute phase.

Chapter 4. Coping with a Repetitive Strain Injury

Important: do not stretch whilst it hurts. If the stretching becomes painful, it is time to stop as you could be causing more damage.

Strengthening exercises are also important for recovering from RSIs, but they are not as simple a matter as stretching. Exercise can cause RSIs or make them worse. That's why you should consult a medical professional before starting or continuing an exercise program if you have RSI symptoms. A physical or occupational therapist, osteopath or chiropractor can prescribe the best exercises for your condition and show you how to do them correctly. RSI-sufferers should exercise under medical guidance which is why this book does not include strengthening exercises.

10. Support Groups

Isolation and depression are two serious concerns for people with RSIs. Support groups for RSI-sufferers are helpful ways to feel connected with other people who share your experiences. They provide information about RSIs as well as different perspectives on treatment, recovery, and coping. RSI-UK (www.rsi-uk.org.uk/) can connect people to online or local support groups. RSI Action (http://www.rsiaction.org.uk/rsi-groups/) lists RSI groups in the U.K. and beyond. Typing Injury FAQ (http://www.tifaq.org/rsi-organisations/rsi-supportinjured-worker-groups.html) lists RSI support groups in the U.S.

11. Journaling

Keeping a journal of RSI symptoms can help you understand what makes you feel better and what makes you feel worse. It can help you to connect the dots between your activities and your symptoms. Journaling also has a psychological benefit; people often feel they have more control over their condition when they journal. By tracking the events and results, symptoms appear less random and less beyond your control.

RSI-sufferer's story. *An active middle aged woman started having pain in her knees. Although she had had RSIs in the past she had never had knee problems before, and couldn't figure out why the pain and tenderness came on all of a sudden. She had kept an RSI diary before, so she decided to write down when she felt the knee pain and what she was doing at the time. It didn't take many entries in her journal for her*

Chapter 4. Coping with a Repetitive Strain Injury

to see that her knees hurt when they bumped the dashboard in her car. (On vacation, when she didn't drive, her knees felt better.) She hadn't changed cars, but she had adjusted her seat forward several weeks earlier. When she moved her seat back, the pain and tenderness in her knees got better until they no longer bothered her. By using her journal she was able to track her pain and figure out what to change to get better.

12. Intimacy

The depression, pain, and physical limitations that often accompany

> **Sex is no fun anymore.**

RSIs can make intimacy difficult, but not necessarily impossible. Some RSI-sufferers report that they feel better after sex.

Here are a number of ideas that can help you enjoy sex when you have RSI.

Communication is always important for intimacy, but even more so when you have an injury. Tell your partner what you can and cannot do, what feels good and what doesn't. He or she can't know what you want or need unless you tell them.

Trust is another issue. Once you have an RSI, it may take time before you and your partner feel comfortable enough to have sex. Be patient, take your time.

Be creative and find new ways to please each other. Positions you used before may not feel good to you, so find others that don't put pressure on your arms. Use your mouth or feet for touching. Try sex toys.

Find advice and encouragement from sex books.

During sex and sleeping make sure you are not in a position that cuts off circulation to your arms and hands.

Sit up to keep the circulation going in your arms and hands.

Warm up the room before you have sex.

If you're not ready for sex, try other ways of being intimate—like gently touching each other's bodies, relaxing, and opening up to your natural feelings.

13. Paying Attention to Emotions

For most people, RSIs bring up a torrent of emotions. People fear losing their livelihoods, relationships, and enjoyment of life. They may see their independence, financial security, and ability to deal with daily life slipping away. It's understandable that they would be upset, angry, depressed, or afraid.

Depression has many faces. You may feel sad, cry easily, and feel helpless. You may have difficulty sleeping, or sleep too much. You may feel guilty, ashamed, or bad about yourself. You may eat more or less, gain weight or lose it. You may become irritable, impatient, or unreasonable without knowing it. Impotence or lack of interest in sex may accompany depression. Friendships may slip away as you isolate yourself. You may use drugs or alcohol to try to relieve the depression—but they only make things worse.

Accepting your injury and the limitations it poses is an important step toward recovery. Acceptance gives your permission to ask for and receive help, starting the process of recovery. The Persian poet Rumi wrote: "If you desire healing, let yourself fall ill."

Feelings can be uncomfortable, especially if you are not used to paying attention to them. You may think having feelings is a sign of weakness, but the truth is that dealing with your emotions is essential to healing. Our emotions are a big part of who we are; we can try to ignore them, or we can learn more about them and use them to support our recovery.

Taking care of your emotions means finding someone you can talk to openly without worrying about judgment or repercussions. That could be a trusted friend, a spiritual counsellor, a support group, or a professional psychotherapist. A medical professional, like a psychiatrist, psychotherapist, or general practitioner, can help you develop a treatment plan for the depression. You may decide to take medication as part of your treatment plan. The plan may include taking

Chapter 4. Coping with a Repetitive Strain Injury

depression medications as well as making changes in your outlook and lifestyle.

A positive attitude, hard as that may seem, aids recovery from depression. Treat yourself kindly, with compassion--as you would a friend who is in pain. Focus on your progress, on small improvements in functioning and pain relief. Stay active, finding hobbies or volunteer work that you enjoy. A repetitive strain injury may limit your activities, but it doesn't eliminate all activities.

In the words of Martin Luther King, Jr.:

"As my sufferings mounted I soon realized that there were two ways in which I could respond to my situation -- either to react with bitterness or seek to transform the suffering into a creative force. I decided to follow the latter course."

14. Finances

RSI-sufferer's story: "I've ...spent money on prescriptions, osteos, ice/ heat packs, massagers, VR software, microphones, acupuncture, Alexander technique lessons etc so we must be talking £3000 plus. I had to work part time for a few months in 2001 because I was ill so I lost around £2,400 in income that year. I've just spent extra money on an automatic car so it's less pressure on my hands so that's another extra cost. I've been lucky though and kept working so I've been able to afford these things. I can't see that someone on sick/ disability pay could." Source: Watson, M. 2009. Investigating the experiences of people with RSI. http://etheses.qmu.ac.uk/133/

RSIs can put a financial strain on families and individuals. In addition to lost wages, there are likely to be expenses for doctors, medications, alternative therapies, assistive devices, and services.

Health insurance may cover some or most of the medical expenses. Most employers in the UK must carry liability insurance, which can cover lost wages and medical expenses for work-related RSIs. In addition, workers with RSIs who belong to unions may be entitled to benefits from them. Directgov (http://www.direct.gov.uk) has information on various disability benefits for which RSI-sufferers may

Chapter 4. Coping with a Repetitive Strain Injury

qualify, including Industrial Injuries Disablement Benefits, Community Care Grants, and others.

RSI-sufferers story: *"Having blown all my wages on remedies, it seems the only real way to alleviate the ailment is to type less, which isn't easy when your entire working existence takes place electronically, you have book deadlines to meet and writing is all you can do."* Source: Freddy Terranean on Henrik Warne's blog, 26 February 2012

15. Service Animals

Most people think of service dogs as guide dogs for people with visual impairments, but these highly trained canines can also help people with other disabilities, such as RSIs. Service dogs, also referred to as assistance dogs, help people with a disability to be as independent and as integrated into society as people without disabilities.

The U.S. American with Disabilities Act of 1990 (ADA) defines a service animal as an animal that has been "individually trained to do work or performs tasks for the benefit of a person with a disability." The ADA defines disability as a "mental or physical condition which substantially limits a major life activity." The "major life activities" include some of the activities people with RSIs have difficulty doing, such as caring for themselves, performing manual tasks, and working.

RSI-sufferer's story: *"It was great to have guests, but it made more work for me. My arms were hurting after tidying up. I just didn't have the energy to carry the linens up the stairs to the guest room, so my dog did it for me. She's a great help."*

Here are just some of the tasks service dogs trained as mobility assistants can do to help people with RSIs:

- Bring objects such as portable phones, medications, beverages, etc... to you.

- Bring in groceries from the car.

- Unload groceries from sacks.

- Pick up dropped items.

Chapter 4. Coping with a Repetitive Strain Injury

- Drag bedding and clothing to the clothes washer.
- Help load the clothes washer.
- Unload clothes dryer.
- Bring clothes.
- Help with dressing and undressing (for example, pulling off socks).
- Help tidy the house or yard by picking up and depositing objects as directed.
- Carry items up or down stairs.
- Bring in mail or newspapers.
- Open and close doors and drawers.
- Push doorbells and elevator buttons.

Service dogs can also be trained to help with less tangible tasks, such as relieving the pain and depression that many RSI-sufferer's experience. Psychiatric service dogs can help by waking up a person who sleeps too much, reminding the person to take medication or eat, find lost items, and give tactile stimulation and comfort through snuggling and petting. Service dogs can help people with RSIs regain their confidence, feel less lonely, and get out into the world.

RSI-sufferer's story: *"I have a service dog for pain and agitation caused by constant pain. Although the pain does not go away, my service dog refocuses my energy away from the negative feelings caused by pain. She also keeps me very active and much more social."* Source: http://lauraschneider.hubpages.com/hub/Why-use-service-dogs-for-invisible-disabilities

16. Returning to Work

The majority of people who take time away from work because of the limitations of RSIs want to return to their jobs. Working is good for most people: it can relieve depression and isolation, stimulate interest, and give purpose to life. However, going back to work is not a simple matter for RSI-sufferers. They may feel pressured to return to their jobs before they are ready—maybe they are afraid they'll lose their jobs if they take too much time off. If their work contributed to their RSI, they can't do the same work under the same conditions anymore otherwise the RSI will just flare up and keep them out of work again. Employers have to be willing to make adjustments to their work. Due to your work limitations you may feel bad about yourself, that you are not carrying your weight. Other people at work may think you are lazy or are getting unfair advantages or even that you are faking your injury. There's a lot to contend with when you return to work, and you must advocate for yourself.

The decision about when you return to work is typically made by you, your doctor, an insurance representative, and your employer or employer's representative. It is important that your doctor understands how much pain and mobility restrictions you have. The better your doctor understands how you feel, the more able he will be to make appropriate recommendations for your return to work.

Your doctor may specify certain conditions under which you can return to work. You and your employer will have to work together to make sure these accommodations work. Some employers are more willing and able than others to accommodate employees who return to work with a repetitive strain injury.

RSI & Overuse Injury Association of the Act Inc (http://www.rsi.org.au/work.html) has a detailed discussion of the topic from the perspective of the worker with a repetitive strain injury.

17. Asking for Help

Many people with RSIs find that they need more help with daily activities than they did before. It seems that the more we need help, the harder it is to ask for it. While we may not hesitate to help a friend, we may feel uncomfortable asking that same friend for help.

Here are some ideas to make asking easier:

- Take advantage of help that you may not have accepted in the past. For example, say yes when the grocery bagger offers to

Chapter 4. Coping with a Repetitive Strain Injury

carry your sacks to your car, or pull up to a petrol station that has attendants to pump for you.

- If you are able to pay for services that will make life easier for you. Send out the ironing and pay a cleaning service to change the bedding and hoover, it will be easier to tend to tasks only you can do, like taking care of your children or performing well on your job or playing a round of golf with a friend.

- Barter for help. Maybe a teenager in the neighbourhood will mow your lawn in exchange for help with schoolwork. Or you could babysit a friend's child whilst the friend does the marketing for both of you.

- Ask for what you need on the job. If you need more breaks or a different chair, work with your boss to arrange it. It's difficult to ask at work but if you don't you may not be able to work at all. Remember, it's to your employer's benefit to keep you safe on the job. A good employer will want to know what you need and how to accommodate it.

RSI-sufferers story: *"You are in a confused state of mind, you don't really know what is happening to you: if you are going to get better or continue to get worse. The focus of your energy is on the pain that you are in and particularly if you haven't got support structures around you and people being assertive on your behalf, you just feel like you are caught in a strong current that you can't get out of."* Source: RSI and Overuse Injury Association of the ACT

Chapter 5. Preventing Repetitive Strain Injuries

RSIs are not inevitable; they don't have to happen. Whether at home or at work, there are many ways to do repetitive tasks and avoid injury, including correct posture, ergonomic workstation design, safer work practices, stretching, and using technology.

1. Computer Workstation Setup

The term "ergonomics" has been thrown around a lot in the past 20 years. Ergonomics is about the relationship between people and the work that they do. Ergonomics focuses on fitting jobs to the people performing them, because when you try the reverse—fitting people to their jobs—you get injuries, illnesses, and errors. By designing workstations properly, ergonomics plays an important role in repetitive strain injury prevention. Ergonomics is also useful for accommodating people with RSIs so they can work without risking further injury.

A poorly arranged workstation makes it difficult to work in a comfortable position. By setting up your workstation correctly, you can make it easier to maintain a safe range of postures.

You don't have to buy new furniture if you can modify what you have to allow comfort and maintain a reasonable posture. The following specifications provide the parameters for a good ergonomic workstation.

Chapter 5. Preventing Repetitive Strain Injuries

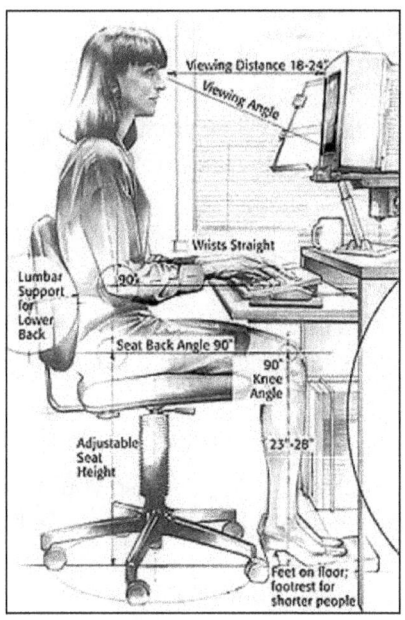

Ergonomic Workstation Setup

(Source: www.ergonomics-info.com)

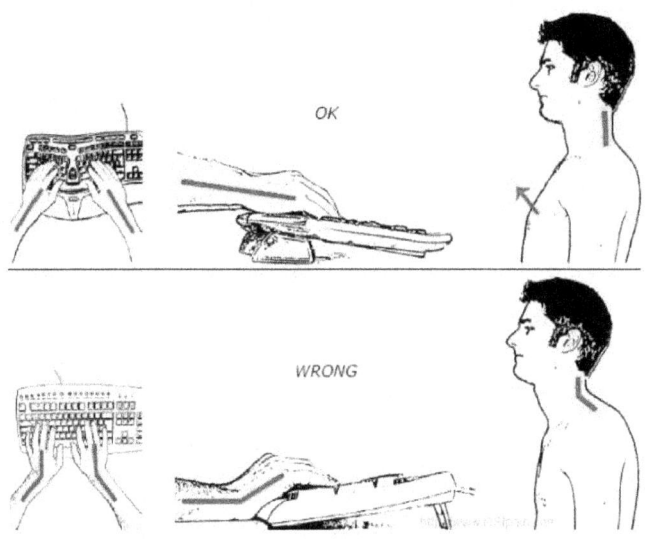

Source : www.rispain.com

Desk Surface

Chapter 5. Preventing Repetitive Strain Injuries

The desk surface needs to be large enough to place the monitor directly in front of you and at least 20 inches away.

An adjustable height desk will allow you to change positions and let other people use the computer comfortably. Sit/stand desks let users change from sitting to standing.

Leave plenty of room under the desk for your legs, feet, and thighs.

If the desk surface has a hard edge, pad the edges (for example, with pipe insulation) to avoid constricting your wrists.

Monitor

Place the monitor directly in front of you so your head, neck and body face directly forward when you look at the screen. If you work mostly from printed documents, place the monitor slightly to the side and keep the printed material in front of you, as close to the monitor as possible. Use a document holder to keep the printed material at the same level as the monitor.

Place the monitor 20-40 inches from the user. You should be able to read text easily with your head and body upright and your back supported by your chair.

Position the top of the screen at or just below eye level. Bifocal users may have to lower the monitor or raise the height of the chair to be able to view the monitor without bending the neck.

Position the monitor at right angles to windows to reduce glare. Glare is where sun light or a light shines on the monitor, making it more difficult to read the text on the monitor. Use an anti-glare screen if necessary.

Another good idea is to use two screens (see picture below) for example, one for your e-mails and the second for other work. This will keep your head and neck from staying in one position all day. All you need is a cable and software to install the second screen. One University professor uses one screen for grading papers and another for everything else. In addition to relieving pressure on her head and neck, this system is more efficient, which means less time on the computer overall. Identical flat screens make the transition from one screen to the other easier.

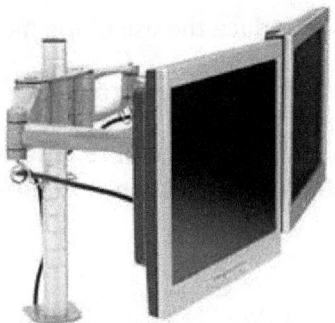

Keyboard

Put the keyboard directly in front of you. Your shoulders should be relaxed and your elbows close to your body, about the same height at the keyboard. Your wrists should be in a neutral position (straight) and in line with your forearms.

Adjust your chair and work surface height as needed to achieve this position. If you cannot adjust them enough, use an adjustable keyboard tray.

If you can afford it, buy an ergonomic keyboard or a split keyboard. Just search for it on the web.

Mouse

Keep the mouse (or other pointing device) close to the keyboard.

Position the mouse/pointer so your wrists can stay in a neutral (that is, straight) position. A wrist or palm rest can help maintain a neutral position.

If the desk or keyboard tray is not large enough for both the keyboard and the mouse, put a mouse tray next to the keyboard tray or a mouse platform above the numeric keypad.

Choose a mouse that fits your hand and that you can use without bending your wrist. Try different types of pointing devices, such as a touchpad, trackball, or fingertip joystick, to find one that is comfortable and suitable for you.

Chapter 5. Preventing Repetitive Strain Injuries

Do not grip the mouse/pointer tightly. Adjust the sensitivity and speed so you can control it with a light touch.

Use keyboard shortcuts to reduce the use of the mouse.

Alternate hands to give each hand a rest from mousing.

If you can afford it, buy an ergonomic mouse, just search for it on the web and you will find loads. Here's just one example:

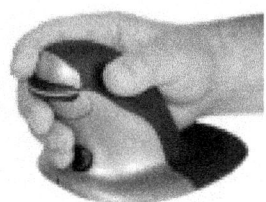

Chair

A good chair for a computer workstation should promote good posture and allow for a range of positions. There's no single chair that's right for everyone, but there are common characteristics of a good ergonomic chair. An adjustable chair offers the most options for positioning for comfort. It's a good idea to try several chairs before selecting one.

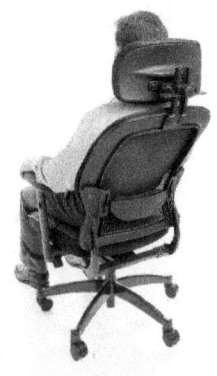
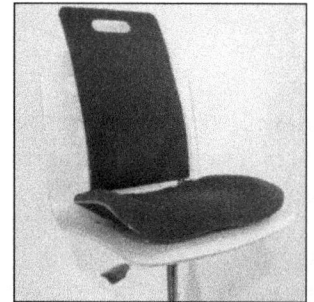

Chapter 5. Preventing Repetitive Strain Injuries

Adjustable office chair with lumbar support and 5-point base and next to it an ergonomic back support that can also help.

Here are the recommendations for a standard ergonomic office chair:

- Seat height. Some "adjustable" chairs are so hard to adjust it's not worth the effort. An easily adjustable chair will have a pneumatic lever that changes the seat height from about 40 to 53 cm from the ground. Your feet should be flat on the floor when sitting in the chair. If you can't adjust the chair so your feet are flat on the floor, use a stable footrest. Many people use a footrest even if their feet reach the floor; it keeps blood circulating in the legs.

- Seat pan. A seat pan (the part you sit on) between 43 and 50 cm wide is good for most users. Larger users may need chairs with larger seat pans. The front to back depth should allow the user to sit against the backrest and have about 7½ cm between the back of the knees and the front of the seat pan. The tilt of the seat pan should be easily adjustable. The seat pan should be padded and have a rounded (waterfall) edge.

- Lumbar support. The lumbar support is in the outward curve of the backrest, which should fit into the small of the back.

- Backrest. The backrest may be separate from the seat or attached to the seat. If it's separate, the height and angle should be adjustable and should lock in place.

- Armrests. Armrests are optional (but not recommended for children). Your arms should not be on the armrests when typing. Armrests should be soft and adjusted to your shoulders so that they relax . Keep your elbow close to your body.

- Base. A five-point base with casters makes the chair stable and easy to move.

Alternative types of office chairs may take some getting used to, but they can be worth the effort, especially for people with lower back pain.

Chapter 5. Preventing Repetitive Strain Injuries

- Ergonomic stool. Ergonomic stools are designed to help computer users sit in a good posture. Stools support the low back and prevent sitting in a hunched position. The seat platform should allow motion in all four directions and should allow the user to sit at the height that is right for him or her.

- Kneeling chair. Sitting in a modified kneeling position with no backrest slides the hips forward and aligns the back, neck, and shoulders. By distributing the weight between the pelvis and knees, this chair relieves the stress on the lower back. The kneeling chair makes it easy to maintain a safe and comfortable posture.

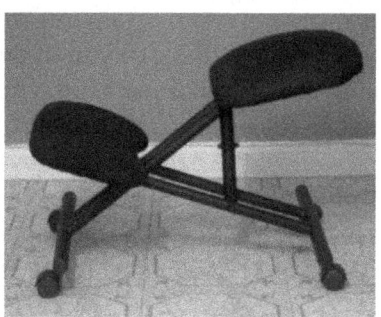

- Kneeling Chair Source: http://upload.wikimedia.org/wikipedia/commons/f/fb/Kneeling_chair.jpg

- Exercise Ball Chair. This unique seat is a big round ball. The slight bouncing of the ball keeps the legs moving, which keeps circulation going and muscles active. Like the kneeling chair, the ball chair encourages proper posture.

2. Posture Matters

What's the first thing that comes into your mind when you think about posture? For a lot of people the first thing they think of is standing ramrod straight without moving—like the guards at Buckingham Palace. Or maybe it's remembering grammar school and being scolded for squirming around in your seat and not sitting straight and still. With images like these it's no wonder many of us don't know what good posture really is—and don't really want to think about it either.

Chapter 5. Preventing Repetitive Strain Injuries

Good posture is about movement, not about being still. Pascarelli and Quilter define good posture as follows: "...good posture really means balanced use of muscles, ease of movement, and freedom from pain, not the tension that comes from holding yourself still...It is the ability to maintain proper alignment of the bones and length of the muscles through movement." Source: Repetitive Strain Injury: A Computer User's Guide

Awkward (or poor or faulty) posture is a major risk factor for repetitive strain injuries. Poor posture stresses the muscles of the neck and shoulder, sending them into spasm. The aggravated muscles can pinch the nerves of the upper body, causing pain and other symptoms.

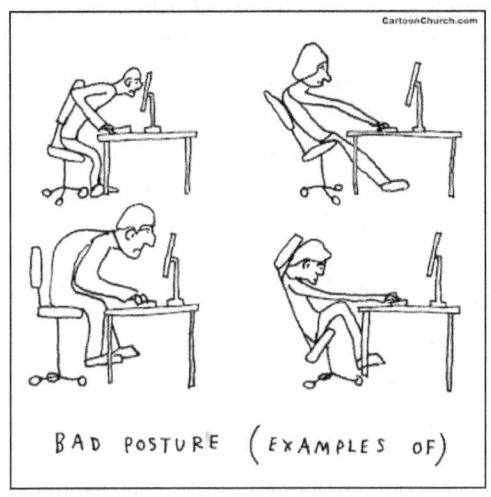

(Source: www.ergonomics-info.com)

Examples of Bad Posture

To understand the importance of the position of your hands when keying, try this: Holding your dominant hand with your thumb on top, grab a thick pen or similar object. Hold your hand in a neutral position (wrist, hand, and fingers in a straight line). Squeeze as tight as you can, then release. Now, grasp the item again and bend your wrist down, so your little finger moves closer to your wrist. (This position is called ulnar deviation.) Now squeeze. Can you feel how much more effort it takes to hold the pen tight? Now try it with your knuckles on top and your wrist bent back (extension), now with your wrist bent forward (flexion).

Most people find that it takes a whole lot more effort to hold onto the pen when the wrist is not in a neutral position, not aligned with the forearm and the hand. This is because the bending pinches the soft tissue and vessels, so it takes more effort. Think of it like a garden hose: when the hose is bent it takes more water pressure to get the same amount of water out. It's that extra effort, over time, that causes the small tears that add up to repetitive strain injuries.

Poor posture is hard to change, especially for people who are not particularly aware of their bodies or have been doing a job for a long time. A perfectly set up computer workstation can help users to hold their bodies properly, but it can't make them do it. Several of the RSI therapies discussed above, particularly the Feldenkrais Method and Alexander Technique, help people become more aware of their bodies and teach them how to put their bodies into alignment. It's not a bad idea to get postural assistance so you don't get a repetitive strain injury, rather than waiting until you do get one.

3. Safer Practices for Computer Users

a) Change your ways
Whether you use the computer for work or pleasure, how you do your computer work makes a big difference. Changing your ways is the first step in preventing injury.

- Vary your activities. Break up the time you spend keyboarding by doing other activities that involve moving around and using different parts of your body. Stand up, take a walk, do something different.

- Get physical exercise. People who are physically active when they are not working have a lower risk of developing RSIs.

- Take regular breaks to reduce eyestrain and muscle strain. Don't work at the computer for more than 40 minutes without a break and break for at least 5-10 minutes every hour. Move around during your break. Timelessness seems to set in when

Chapter 5. Preventing Repetitive Strain Injuries

working on the computer; it's easy to lose track of time. That's where break reminder software comes in—in case you forget, it reminds you. www.breakremindersoftware.com

- Look away from the monitor frequently and focus your eyes on a distant object. This gives the eyes a chance to relax and helps prevent eyestrain. It only takes three hours a day in front of the computer to develop symptoms of computer vision syndrome, especially dry eyes and eye fatigue.

b) Typing technique
Proper typing technique is neither common sense nor intuitive; it has to be learned. Keep wrists straight when typing or using a mouse. The neutral (straight) position is with the wrist parallel to the floor and the middle finger at the middle of the wrist.

Don't rest elbows, wrists or forearms on the desk or wrist rest whilst typing or using a mouse. Wrists should float above the surface whilst typing. They can rest on the surface when not typing.

Don't stretch fingers to reach keys. Instead, let the shoulders and arms move the fingers over the keyboard.

Keep fingers curved. Fingernails have to be short to keep the fingers curved while keying. Don't hold the thumb or little finger in the air.

Touch type. Use the lightest possible touch when typing or using the mouse. Don't pound or press.

Hold the mouse loosely with all fingers. Don't grip or grasp tightly and don't raise the little finger.

4. The Problem with Sitting
Too much sitting is bad for your health. New research has found that excessive sitting may lead to obesity, type 2 diabetes, and heart disease. According to the American Cancer Society, women who sit for more than six hours a day are 37 percent more likely to die prematurely. Men are 18 percent more likely to die early if they sit too much. Medical professionals have long known that staying in one position for too long contributes to RSIs.

Chapter 5. Preventing Repetitive Strain Injuries

Furthermore, research concludes that vigorous exercise does not make up for long periods of sitting. That is, if you sit all day and then work out at the gym, you are still vulnerable to all the negative consequences of your sedentary day. Experts recommend frequent short breaks during the day to offset the sitting—active breaks where you move around. You don't have to stop working, just stop sitting.

Human bodies are built to move; when they don't, they suffer. Sitting causes the central nervous system to slow down, which leads to fatigue and sluggishness. Sitting weakens muscles and stiffens joints and as a result, posture gets distorted and the back and joints hurt.

When you sit at a desk typing, some of your muscles work too much and some work too little. This can result in painful muscles when you get off your chair or when you wake up in the morning. In just a short time of sitting, the body's electrical activity and blood circulation drop significantly. You can lose the ability to move. The body's effective use of insulin quickly goes down by 40 percent. The body burns calories at one-third its normal rate; just standing up triples the body's energy use. It doesn't take long for sitting to take its toll on the body.

James Levine, MD, PhD is an endocrinologist at the Mayo Clinic. He is responsible for some of the groundbreaking work on the effects of sitting, and concluded: "Excessive sitting is a lethal activity." Dr. Levine recommends standing desks because they let users make more small movements during the day than is possible when seated. You can buy a standing desk, but it's not hard to make one out of shelves or other furniture.

Dr. Levine designed (and uses) a treadmill desk, where the computer user walks at a very slow speed whilst working on a desk that surrounds the treadmill. Steelcase (http://www.steelcase.com) sells treadmill desks; Treadmill Desk (www.treadmill-desk.com/) has instructions for building your own.

Dr. Levine recommends lots of short, slow speed walks during the day. Here are simple ideas for incorporating walks into the workday:

- Stand up to talk on phone.

Chapter 5. Preventing Repetitive Strain Injuries

- Hold walking meetings. Walking meetings work best with two or three people and when there's no need to take notes.

- Talk to people in person. Walk over to co-workers to deliver messages.

- Make a walking track in the office. Outline a path with tape affixed to the floor.

- Take the stairs.

- Park away from the office; don't take the closest spot.

- Take a midday walk, saving half of your break time for eating lunch and half for walking.

- Use a standing desk or sit/stand desk.

RSI-sufferer's story: I work at home on a laptop and have been having constant pain between the shoulder blades for some time, despite having an adjustable chair, and despite doing my best to sit up straight. Today I put my laptop on a cupboard - about waist height and added a couple of books to raise it a bit more. So far, it is a massive improvement. (From Fishing Genet, commenting on a Guardian article at http://www.guardian.co.uk/society/us-news-blog/2012/jul/10/scientists-sitting-is-bad-for-you)

5. Stretches for Computer Users

Stretching helps to relax your muscles, so they are less likely to get injured. It also breaks up scar tissue that forms from RSIs, which promotes healing. Stretches feel good to most people, and re-energize them. Stretching should not hurt; never stretch to the point of pain. If these stretches are painful, you may already have an injury and should consult your doctor.

The Canadian Centre for Occupational Health and Safety recommends stretches like the following for computer users.

Chapter 5. Preventing Repetitive Strain Injuries

Shoulder Shrug

Raise the top of your shoulders toward your ears until you feel slight tension in your neck and shoulders. Hold for 3-5 seconds. Relax your shoulders and repeat 3 times.

Shoulder Roll 1

Sit down and make yourself as tall as possible. Slowly roll your shoulder to the back in a circular motion. Then roll your shoulders forward. Repeat 5 times each way.

Shoulder Roll 2

Stand up and put your hands at your side and relax your shoulders. Slowly roll your shoulders in a backwards and forewords direction and try to make the circle you make by rolling as large as possible. Repeat 5 times each way.

Shoulder Stretch

Sit down on a chair and put your hands behind your heads with your elbows pointing outwards. Push your elbows gently forward towards each other and try to stretch until the tips of your elbows touch. Hold for 5 seconds and repeat a few times.

Neck Stretcher 1

Drop your head slowly to the left, trying to touch your left shoulder with your left ear until you feel the stretch in the right side of your neck. Hold for 3 seconds Bring your head back to normal position. Drop your head slowly to the right, trying to touch your right shoulder with your right ear until you feel the stretch in the left side of your neck. Hold for 3 seconds. Bring your head back to normal position. Repeat 3 times each way.

Neck Stretcher 2

Drop your head slowly to the left, trying to touch your left shoulder with your left ear . Then, slowly drop your chin to your chest; turn your

Chapter 5. Preventing Repetitive Strain Injuries

head all the way to the left, then all the way to the right. You should feel the stretch in your neck. Repeat 3 times and do the other side.

Neck Stretcher 3

Turn your head sideways as far as comfortable as you are looking to the left. Bend your neck over to look at the floor until you feel a stretch. Hold for 3 seconds. Return your head in original position and do the other side. Repeat 3 times.

Wrist Turns

Sit down and put your arms next to you. Turn your arms and wrist so that your palm faces outwards away from your body and then back inwards. Feel the stretch in your lower arm. Hold for 3 seconds. Repeat 3 times.

Upper Arm Stretcher

Sit down or stand up. Put your right arm forwards with the palm facing the floor. Now put your left hand underneath your right elbow and turn the palm of your right hand facing towards the left. With your left arm pull your right arm towards you so you can feel the stretch in your right upper arm. Hold for 3 seconds. Repeat 3 times with each arm.

Head turns

Drop your head down towards your chest as far as it feels comfortable. Turn your head left trying to look at your left upper arm and hold for 2 seconds. Turn your head right trying to look at your right upper arm and hold for 2 seconds. Repeat 5 times each side.

Back Curl and Leg Stretch

Hold onto your right shin with your right hand. Lift your right leg off the floor. Bend forward, curling your back, and bring your nose toward your knee. Repeat with the other leg.

Leg Stretcher

Sit on a chair and make yourself as tall as possible. Stretch one leg forwards and try to point your toes as far as possible towards you and

Chapter 5. Preventing Repetitive Strain Injuries

hold for 5 seconds. You should feel the stretch throughout your whole leg. Repeat with the other leg. Do 3 times for each leg.

Forward lean

Sit on a chair and put your elbows and arms on your thighs and let your hands relax. Lean your head downwards. Sit like that and take 4 to 5 breaths and return in the sitting position.

Trunk Stretcher (the part of your body between your neck and your waist)

Sit on a chair and make yourself as tall as possible. Drop your arms by your side. Move your left hand towards the floor as far as you can but make sure that your trunk stays upright. Hold your arm for 5 seconds. Return to sitting position and repeat with right arm. Repeat with each arms 3 times.

Forearm Twist

Sit down on a chair and put your hands on your lap with the palms facing your legs. Relax your shoulders. Turn your hands so that your palm is now facing up. Gently push your thumbs outwards as far as comfortable and hold for 3 seconds. Turn your hand again to face your legs. Repeat with 5 times.

Stretch your arms and fingers

Sit on a chair and make yourself as tall as possible. Put both of your arms forwards with the palm of your hands facing you. Interlink your fingers. Roll your palms/arms so that they now face away from you. Stretch by reaching out as far as you can and hold for 5 seconds. Feel the stretch in lower arm and fingers. Repeat 3 times.

Stretch your arms and shoulders

Sit on a chair and make yourself as tall as possible. Put both of your arms forwards with the palm of your hands facing you. Interlink your fingers. Roll your palms/arms so that they now face away from you. Move your arms so they are now above your head. Stretch by reaching out as far as you can and hold for 5 seconds. Repeat 3 times.

Chapter 5. Preventing Repetitive Strain Injuries

6. Prevention through Technology

Repetitive motions from using the keyboard and mouse and awkward postures are major contributors to RSIs. You can use features of your computer as well as ergonomically designed equipment to reduce keystrokes and mouse use and eliminate awkward postures.

a) Computer Features

Slow down the mouse to reduce muscle tension in the hand. In Control Panel, double-click on Mouse. Select Pointer Options. Under Pointer Speed, move the slider to the left to Slow. Click OK.

Reduce the number of clicks needed. From the Tools menu select Folder Options. On the General tab find 'Click items as follows' and choose 'Single click to open an item.'

Use keyboard shortcuts to reduce keystrokes and mouse use. To see shortcut keys, go to View/Toolbars/Customise/Options and click on 'show shortcut tips.'

Use AutoCorrect to reduce keystrokes. AutoCorrect not only corrects mistakes, it can also insert phrases and paragraphs you use frequently. Go to Tools/AutoCorrect. Add mistakes you commonly make and the corrections. You can also add phrases and assign them a shortcut phrase. For example, if you have a standard closing paragraph you use for letters, you can add that in AutoCorrect and give it a name, like "closing." Then all you have to type is "closing" and AutoCorrect types the rest.

b) Software

Voice recognition software allows you to operate your computer using just your voice. With hands-free computing your voice turns speech into text, so you don't have to use a keyboard or mouse. Dragon Naturally Speaking (http://www.dragonvoicerecognition.com/) and Talking Desktop (www.talkingdesktop.com/) are popular voice recognition software programs. Some Internet providers offer text-to-speech technology for reading and responding to email.

Break reminder software reminds you take a break if you go too long without one. Examples include www.breakremindersoftware.com, www.workpace.com

Chapter 5. Preventing Repetitive Strain Injuries

c) Hardware

Alternative keyboards use various designs to help users keep their wrists straight, reducing their risk for RSIs. Split keyboards aim to straighten the wrists. Tented keyboards reduce the rotation of the forearms. Adjustable negative slope keyboards keep the hands from bending too far.

Before buying an alternative keyboard, make sure it is compatible with your computer. Then, try the keyboard for a few weeks before you decide if it works for you; it takes a week or two to get used to the differences.

The Goldtouch keyboard is a split keyboard that allows the user to position each section individually for maximum comfort. The Ergostars Saturnus keyboard is compact and easy to carry. You can learn more about these and other ergonomic keyboards at Keytools (http://www.keytools.co.uk/keyboards/) and at ErgonomicKeyboards.org (http://www.ergonomickeyboards.org/).

FrogPad (www.frogpad.com) is a wireless, Bluetooth, one-handed external keyboard that can be used with laptops, PDAs, and mobile phones. External and wireless, you can set the handheld or laptop at the right heights and angles.

Alternative mice relieve the awkward hand positions of most computer mice. A mouse shaped like a joystick is used vertically, positioning the hand more comfortably. Mice of different sizes fit larger and smaller hands. An ergonomic mouse supports the wrist in a neutral position. New designs in trackballs make them easier to use for people without fine motor skills. Keytools (http://www.keytools.co.uk/mice/), gizmag (http://www.gizmag.com/), and The Human Solution (http://www.thehumansolution.com/mice.html) offer selections of ergonomic mice, including hands' free mice for carpal tunnel syndrome sufferers.

Headmouse Extreme is a wireless head-pointing device that translates movements of the head into movements of the mouse. Designed for people who cannot use their hands, it is available from Liberator (http://www.liberator.co.uk/headmouse-extreme.html) and Techcess

Chapter 5. Preventing Repetitive Strain Injuries

(http://www.techcess.co.uk/5_1_headmouse.php) . A programmable foot-controlled mouse (also called slipper mouse) takes all the pressure off the hands; sold through Amazon.com (http://www.amazon.co.uk/Foot-Mouse-Slipper-Programmable-Pedal/dp/B0061DVAOK) and Price Selector (http://uk.price-selector.net/search/foot%20pedal%20mouse?campid=5336926831).

Smartphones. Some newer models open up to a colour monitor and QWERTY keyboard that makes it easier to type with just two or three fingers.

PDA Stylus. Bigger styluses for PDAs are easier to grip. Papermate makes a 3-way pen/pencil/PDA stylus with a padded grip.

Sit/Stand Workstations. Workstations that let workers easily change from a sitting position to a standing position are becoming increasingly popular in schools, offices, and call centres. Ergotron (www.ergotron.com), GeekDesk (www.geekdesk.com/), and Nielsen (www.nielsen-associates.co.uk/sit-stand/) are three of many designers and manufacturers of height adjustable and sit/stand desks.

Scanners. Using a scanner is a practical and efficient way to reduce the amount of typing you have to do. You will need a scanner that has built in OCR software (Optical Character Recognition). All you do is scan a page and it recognises all the characters and brings up the page into MsWord.

Chapter 6. Risk Assessment

1. Identifying Hazards and Risks

Risk assessment involves identifying hazards (things that can cause harm), the chances of being injured or made ill by the hazards, and the seriousness of the potential harm. Risk assessment is an important tool for preventing RSIs and for finding the factors that need to change in order to improve the situation for RSI sufferers. By examining what and how an individual is doing a task, it is possible to make the right adjustments.

Risk assessment is a continuous process. Here's a four-step method for assessing and controlling risks:

1. **Identify hazards**: Think about what you are doing and identify anything that could lead to RSIs. Review your workstation design and safer work practices to find out if your equipment and the way you are using it may lead to RSIs. Think about your posture and how much time you spend on your computer. Employers should ask their employees what they think the risks and hazards are in their jobs.

2. **Assess**. Decide what to do: Decide what you can do to change the hazards you have found. Prioritize the hazards, focusing on those that are most likely to cause serious harm. Then, consider if you can modify your workstation, take more breaks, change your posture, or use software or computer functions to reduce your risk of getting injured.

3. **Act**. Reduce the hazards. Make the changes you decided on. You may be able to make some of the changes right away, like using reams of paper to raise the monitor or taking more breaks. Some of the improvements may cost money, like buying a new mouse or chair.

4. **Monitor the changes**. Pay attention to how you feel after you improve your situation. Do you feel more/less aches, pains, or stress? How comfortable are you? Do your symptoms worsen or get better? You may need to start the assessment process over again if the changes don't create the improvements you

Chapter 6 . Risk Assessment

want. Record your findings.

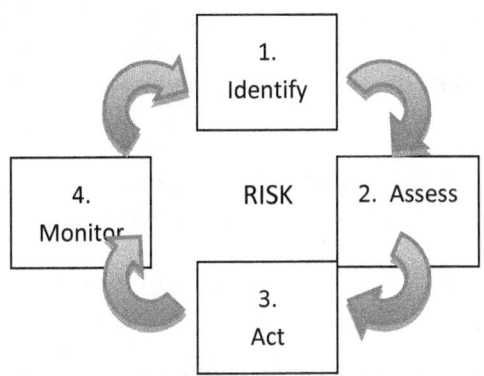

RSI-sufferer's story: *Pat is a government employee who works in a large office. She spends much of the day on her computer. One day, she started feeling pain in her arms and neck. She asked her co-worker to help her figure out why she was having pain all of a sudden, when she hadn't had any problems in the past. Using the assessment process, they discovered that Pat's working surface was too high. They realized that when new furniture was installed throughout the office the previous week, all the work surfaces were set at the same height. As Pat is shorter than most people, her desk was too high, so she was working with her neck bent to see the monitor and her wrists bent to reach the keys. Once her desk was adjusted to the right height for her, all of Pat's symptoms disappeared.*

2. Computer Workstation Checklist

Checklists are easy-to-use assessment tools. The following checklist for computer workstations is adapted from the U.S. Occupational Safety and Health Administration (OSHA). Use it to find out if your workstation is set up properly. For any item you cannot check off, refer to the Computer Station Setup section for ideas on correcting the situation.

Posture

- Head, neck, and torso are upright—not bent down or back.

- Head, neck, and torso face forward—not twisted.

Chapter 6 . Risk Assessment

- Shoulders and upper arms are in line with the torso, about perpendicular to the floor and relaxed –not raised or stretched forward.

- Upper arms and elbows are close to the body—not extended forward.

- Forearms, wrists, and hands are straight and in line, with the forearm at about 90 degrees to the upper arm.

- Wrists and hands are straight—not bent up, down, or sideways.

- Thighs are parallel to the floor with lower legs perpendicular to the floor. Thighs may be raised slightly above knees.

- Feet rest flat on the floor or on a stable footrest.

Chair

- Backrest provides support for lower back (lumbar area)

- Seat pan is the right size for the user.

- Seat front does not press against the back of the knees and lower legs.

- Seat is cushioned, with a rounded front—no sharp edges.

- Armrests, if used, support both forearms and do not interfere with movement.

Keyboard and Mouse

- Surface is stable and large enough to hold a keyboard and mouse (or other input device).

- Input device is right next to the keyboard so it can be used without reaching.

- Input device is easy to use and fits the hand

- Wrists or hands do not rest on sharp edges.

Chapter 6 . Risk Assessment

Monitor

- Top of the screen is at or slightly below eye level, so it can be read without bending the head or neck.

- Monitor is at a distance so you don't have to lean your head, neck, or torso backward or forward to read the screen.

- Monitor is positioned directly in front of user—no twisting of the head or neck needed to see the monitor.

- Glare is not reflected on the screen.

- Screen is free of dirt and dust.

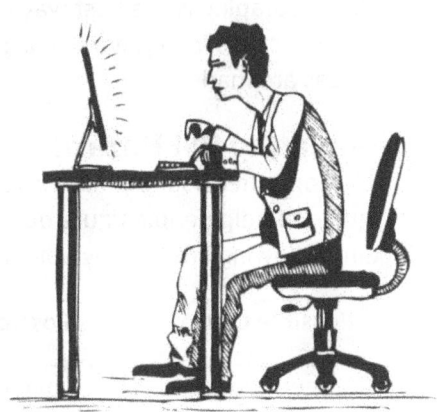

Head and neck bent forward because screen is too far away

Work Area

- Top of thighs have enough clearance under the work surface.

- Legs and feet have enough clearance under the work surface to allow user to get close enough to the keyboard and input device.

General

Chapter 6 . Risk Assessment

- Workstation and equipment can be adjusted so user can change positions and be safe and comfortable.

- Workstation has enough space to access needed supplies and documents without reaching.

- Computer tasks are organized to allow alternating with other tasks as well as adequate breaks.

3. Videotape Assessment
Another way to assess the dangers of repetitive motion is to videotape a person doing the work. Videotaping is the best way to see exactly what you are doing that could cause injury. It's also a great way to see improvements after changes are made.

4. Finding and Eliminating RSI Hazards
Repetitive Strain Injury: A Computer User's Guide has a repetitive strain troubleshooting guide to help people figure out what they are doing to cause them pain. Following are the key points:

Problem	Possible Cause	Possible Remedy
Headache, neck pain	Screen too high	Lower screen
	Spectacles not right for computer work	Get new prescription
	Muscle tension	Relax, stretch
Overall neck pain	Chin jutting forward	Massage, stretch, tuck chin in
Pain on one side of neck	Monitor to the side, not in front	Move monitor in front
Pain in elbow	Table too high, overuse	Lower table, take breaks, work slower, stretch, strengthen

		muscles
Pain on top of forearm, little finger side	Typing with fingers flat, holding little finger up while typing, bending wrists to left or right	Keep fingernails short and wrists straight, technique retraining
Pain in fingertips	Pounding keyboard	Use light touch
Pain in thumb or thumb side of wrist	Overuse, holding thumb up while typing, hitting space bar too hard.	Breaks, use fingers for space bar, technique retraining
Pain on bottom of forearm	Overuse, hands bent down from wrists	Breaks, stretching, massage, posture retraining
Numbness in fingers, pain in wrists	Resting wrists on edge of desk or wrist rest, edge of desk cutting into wrists	Don't rest wrists whilst typing

Chapter 7. Dangers of Laptops

1. Laptop Hazards

> **I can't hold down a job. I don't know if I'll ever be able to work again.**

Laptop computers present particular risks for RSIs. Laptops (or notebooks or tablets) were designed for short term, occasional use; they were not designed to be a computer user's primary computer. With attached keyboards and monitors, there's very little adjustability, making it almost impossible to position a laptop ergonomically.

The common posture for laptop users is with the head bent forward, which puts tremendous strain on the neck. Forward head posture (FHP) reduces lung capacity and impairs digestion. It also flattens the natural curve of the neck, resulting in compression of the spinal discs and an early onset of arthritis. A typical adult head weighs about 5 kg, but when the head is bent it exerts an extra 14 kg of pressure on the spine. To see for yourself, hold a 2-3 kg weight close to your body. Then, still holding onto the weight, extend your arm all the way out. Notice how much heavier the weight feels when it is away from your body.

Frequent, long-term use of laptops causes:

- Neck pain, headaches, and eyestrain from viewing the screen at an awkward angle.

- Wrist and hand problems from bent wrists and overuse of input devices such as roller balls, track balls, and mice.

- Shoulder and back pain from using the laptop whilst in a slouching or bending posture or when lying down.

- Shoulder and back pain from carrying a heavy laptop case, especially if you carry it on one shoulder.

Chapter 7. Dangers of Laptops

- Neck pain and headaches from bending the neck forward.

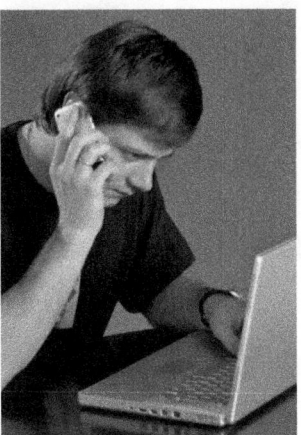

Forward head posture (neck bent) with laptop.

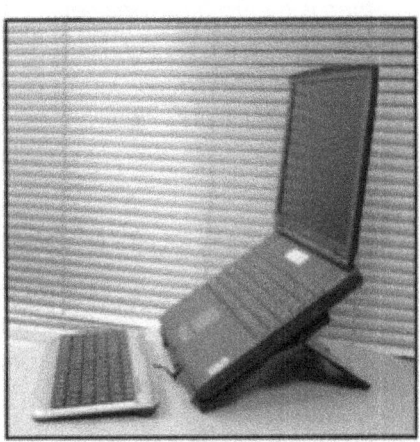

This is an ideal set up for using your laptop so your neck is not always bend forwards. Source: www.laptopstands.co.uk

Chapter 7. Dangers of Laptops

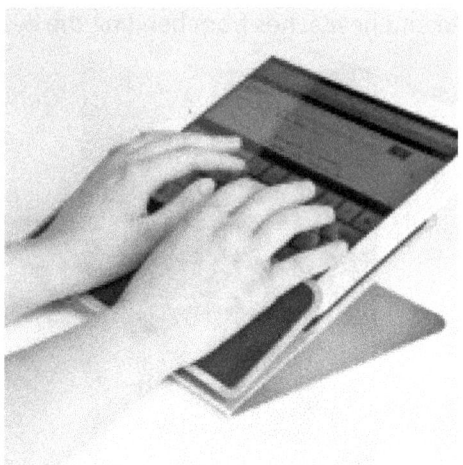

A solution for using your tablet. Source: www.laptopstands.co.uk

RSI-sufferer's story. *John is a journalist. He spends most of his time on location and writes his stories on his laptop. Work was picking up for John; he was excited about his projects, but he started getting severe headaches; the more work he received, the more headaches he got. When he should have been in the field interviewing people for his stories, he was in bed with ice packs on his head.*

At first, John tried to ignore the headaches. When that didn't work he made up reasons for the headaches: it was the food he ate or the pillow he used. When he ran out of excuses and couldn't afford to miss any more time from work he went to a doctor. After asking John about his work the chiropractor suggested that the headaches might be because of the way he works on his computer.

Being an investigative journalist, John had no trouble finding out about the hazards of spending too much time working on a laptop. However, John did not make any changes. Eventually he had to cut back on his work because of the headaches; his career suffered, as did his family life.

Chapter 7. Dangers of Laptops

2. Safer Laptop Practices

Take frequent breaks from your laptop. Look away from your screen, get up, and move around. Stretch your arms, shrug your shoulders, and move your fingers around to relax the muscles. The British Chiropractic Association recommends that you change position at least every 40 minutes.

3. Laptop Setup for Occasional Use

Here's how to set up your laptop for short-term use when you are away from your desktop computer.

- Sit in a comfortable upright chair. Your legs should be at an approximate right angle with your thighs. Put a towel or small pillow behind your lower back for lumbar support.

- Place the laptop on your lap. If you need an adjustment to keep your wrists in a neutral position (that is, straight), try putting an empty 3-ring binder under the laptop with the wide edge toward your knees. (The binder will also keep the heat of the laptop away from your body. But don't put the laptop on top of a pillow because that can interfere with the computer's fan.)

4. Laptop Setup for Long-term Use

Whilst laptops lack the ergonomic features needed for safe keying over an extended period of time, the reality is that many people use laptops as their primary computers. If you're in that category, here's how to set up your laptop to reduce your risk for RSIs.

- Place your laptop on an adjustable table or desk or an adjustable keyboard tray. A laptop desk or stand (http://www.laptopstands.co.uk/) may be the perfect solution.

- Adjust the surface so the top of the laptop monitor at or slightly below eye level. If you don't have an adjustable surface, use reams of paper on a stationary table or desk to raise or lower your laptop.

- Angle the screen so you don't have to bend your head forward;

Chapter 7. Dangers of Laptops

- Place the screen at a right angle to windows and away from overhead lighting to minimise glare. If you need more light use a laptop light plugged into a USB port;

- Make sure your shoulders, feet and knees all face the same direction;

- Clean the screen frequently with an anti-static cleaner safe for laptops. Dust can make it hard to read the screen, increasing eyestrain and the tendency to bend your head forward;

- Use a document holder to hold documents vertically and at the same height as the screen. This reduces neck strain from having to look down at documents.

- Attach a regular size external keyboard to the laptop so you can work with your hands in a neutral position (that is, with wrists straight). Put the keyboard on an adjustable desk or keyboard tray, positioned at or just below elbow height.

Another good idea is to use a docking station whenever possible.

5. How to Choose a Laptop

To reduce the risk for RSI, look for these features when buying a laptop:

- Light weight, no more than 3 kg;

- 35 cm diagonal screen, or larger;

- Keys as large as possible;

- Detachable or height adjustable screen if available;

- Long battery life so you don't have to carry cables;

- Touch pad, roller ball or external mouse rather than a track point pointing device;

- Tilt adjustable keyboard;

Chapter 7. Dangers of Laptops

- Mechanism for attaching external mouse, external monitor, or numeric keypad.

6. How to Carry a Laptop Safely

When you add in the weight of the case, cords, and accessories, a laptop is not so light. Carrying a heavy laptop case on one shoulder puts tremendous strain on your shoulder, neck, and back. There are safer ways to carry your laptop.

Rucksacks distribute the weight better than shoulder bags. Choose a rucksack with well-padded shoulder and waist straps. Carry the rucksack on both shoulders and adjust the straps so the rucksack stays close to your back.

A wheeled carrying case is another good option. Make sure the handle is long enough so you don't have to stoop. It's easier on your back if you push, rather than pull, the wheeled case.

If you must use a single strap bag, choose a lightweight one with a long handle so you can carry it messenger bag style, with the strap over one shoulder and the bag under the other arm.

BBP Bags (http://bbpbags.com/) makes backpack and messenger style carrying cases. Bizrate (http://www.bizrate.co.uk/computercases_bags/products_keyword--rolling+computer+bag.html) carries a selection of wheeled, rucksack, and messenger style bags.

RSI-sufferer's story. *Dr. John P said:*

After my surgeries, the orthopedic surgeon told me if I worked on a regular computer again I would become paralyzed from the neck down.

I am 66 and have been going through this since 1991 and have tried nearly 100 medications and the results are and have always been ... fair to none, narcotics shut off pain, but label you in the eyes of everyone, and they don't judge fairly - and nsaids are useless and dangerous. Steroids have their own issue and continued use causes dowager's hump - pretty ugly.

Chapter 7. Dangers of Laptops

There are unique pills that reduce pain, but the next day pain is 5x worse (side effects are worse). (all non-narcotic)
There are steroid shots - reduce pain for 24-36 hours.

Instead I use a laptop and my diagnosis is - osteoarthritis of the hands and fingers, osteoporosis of the fingers and joints, and tendonitis - all verified by film. **This is after 17 years on laptops.**

I am looking for a cure, because here there is no surgery or treatment for this ailment. **My RSI is so bad that I cannot turn the key in the car to open doors or start the engine. My hands don't work like that anymore.**
I order TIGER BALM - from Thailand, 12 bottles at a time, last me over a year and I massage it into my neck (surgery 1994- fusion, bore spur remains, constant pain) and I do neck rolls, and shoulder shrugs, tense and release exercises and sleep on a memory foam pillow: 4 of them. For my hands - which are very sad, I eat Jello (gelatin) - and take NSAIDS but the pain never leaves.
Cold/ice helps the hands, hot and warm helps the neck.

The best thing I have is a home made snake 6" diameter about 1 meter long, filled with old corn, old beans also works - but it must be stale and non-edible. Otherwise problems.
I have had 33 surgeries as a result of allowing US surgeons to work on my neck and back ... and I am now able to walk 1 block, most of the time is in a chair or memory foam bed ... I cannot travel, take vacations, and the prognosis is 2-3 years until I can't walk.

Chapter 8. Cell Phones, Video Games and Other Hand Held Devices

1. The Hazards

With 93.5 million text messages being sent every day in the UK, RSIs from texting could become an epidemic. In response to a question on Yahoo, one texter said she sent over 8,000 text messages in one month (that's over 250 a day)! London-based Virgin Mobile reports that 38 percent of its frequent users have sore thumbs and wrists from texting. That's not all: each year 3.8 million people experience an injury related to texting.

Video games are a billion dollar industry with the amazing graphics and music but obviously from a commercial point of view the video games manufacturers are not telling you that overuse can affect your future.

Playing video games usually means hours of immobility and this prevents proper blood flow to the extremities. The spine can be curved unnaturally and become very painful as most people play games with a curved back.

Cell phones, video game consoles, and other hand held devices haven't been around long enough to see the kinds of long term problems they might cause. However, short-term health effects are becoming common enough to have their own names. "Text messaging injury" or "TMI" is pain and swelling of tendons at the base of the thumb and the wrists. It's common amongst young adults as well as working people who are tied to their jobs via texting. "Cell phone elbow" refers to pain, tingling, and numbness in the arm and forearm from bending the arm for long periods of time.

Texting Thumb, Nintendo Thumb or Nintendinitis are now terms used often in the medical industry.

Chapter 8. Cell Phones, Video Games Other Hand Held Devices

> **I had to cut my hair short because it hurt too much to brush my long hair.**

Looking at a typical handheld device, it's easy to see how it could cause a repetitive strain injury. The small size requires a tight grip, as does the tiny stylus of most PDAs. As the screen is so small, users hunch over to see it, bending their necks, stooping their shoulders, and rounding their backs. Clenching a phone between the ear and the shoulder requires even more neck bending. In fact, neck pain is the most common complaint of frequent cell phone users. Thumbing messages repeats the same small motions over and over resulting in TSI.

A study conducted in Taiwan measured the changes the body goes through during texting. Eighty-three percent of the study participants reported hand and neck pain whilst they were texting; plus, they held their breath when they received text messages.

2. Safer Use of Mobile Phones

You can reduce the risk of getting a RSI from a hand held device by paying attention to these safe practices:

- Hold the device in one hand and use the fingers of the other hand to type. Don't hold it in one hand and use the thumb of that hand for keying.

- Store commonly used numbers in the cell phone's address book to reduce the amount of keying you have to do.

- Use a headset for phone calls, or hold the phone in your hand.

- Switch sides every 10 minutes if you must cradle the phone between your ear and shoulder.

- Limit your texting to no more than 1½ hours in 24 hours.

- Use handheld devices for short messages only.

- If your hands start to hurt, stop texting and massage your arm from wrist to elbow.

Chapter 8. Cell Phones, Video Games Other Hand Held Devices

- Change position frequently and stretch your arms, shrug your shoulders, and move your fingers around to relax your muscles.

- Try out new hand held devices before you buy them to make sure you can use them comfortably.

- Use the predictive text feature of the mobile phone to reduce keystrokes.

- Keep your shoulders relaxed, down away from your ears. Bring the device into your field of sight rather than bending your body to see it. Hold the device below the level of your heart and keep your back straight.

- When using a device for tasks other than phone calls, keep elbows next to your body, bent at about 135 degrees. Keep your head straight and over your shoulders. Look down on the device without bringing your head forward.

3. Safer Use of Video games

There is no need to totally give up the fun of video games but here are some important tips that will help to prevent injury:

- Don't sit with a "hunched back". However uncomfortable it may feel at the beginning try and sit with a straight back.

- Just like the athletes warm up their muscles, it is important that you warm up your hands before starting to game. If you are playing electronic tennis, warm up your arms and elbows. Basically warm up the body parts you will be using most whilst gaming.

- Don't put your hands very tightly around the controller as this can over tighten the tendons. Instead, hold the controller as light as possible in your hands and push the buttons gently (however excited you are getting with the game).

- Take regular breaks. I spoke to teenagers who literally spend 3 hours on a game without any breaks! That is a Definite No!

Chapter 8. Cell Phones, Video Games Other Hand Held Devices

- Pause the game at least every 30 minutes and go for a short walk have a drink, stretch your legs, etc.. just move!

- Do some stretches on a regular basis - every 10 to 15 minutes or so. Just stretch your arms and legs forwards, raise your arms over your head, move your shoulders up and down.

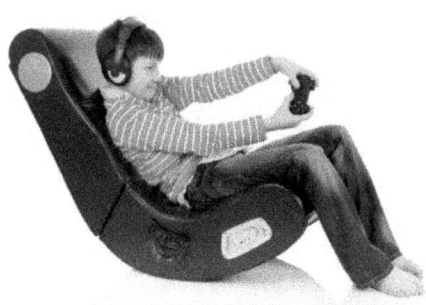

An ergonomic gaming chair is ideal to use when playing games. Much better than "hunching" on the bed.

4. Stretches for Texters

Virgin Mobile and the British Chiropractic Association suggest stretches to reduce the risk of repetitive strain injury amongst people who are heavy texters. Use these exercises before and after texting and between texts if you are doing it for long periods of time. These stretches should not hurt. If they do, it's time to seek medical advice.

Thumb stretch

With the right palm facing down, hold the thumb of the right hand with the fingers of the left hand. Pull the thumb gently and hold for 10 seconds. Repeat three times, then reverse hands.

Arm stretch

Stretch your left arm in front of you, palm up. Place your right hand on top of the left with fingers and thumbs lined up. Point your fingers down and hold for 10 seconds. You should feel a gentle stretch on the inside of your left forearm/wrist. Repeat three times, then reverse hands.

Finger stretch

Hold hand out, palm down. Spread fingers and thumbs as far as you can. Hold 2-3 seconds. Then make a fist and hold 2-3 seconds. Repeat 3 times.

Arm and finger stretcher

Sit in a chair and make yourself as tall as possible. Lean back as far as you can so you are looking towards the ceiling. Spread your arms (like you did as a kid when you were flying an aeroplane) and rotate your arms left and right. Spread your fingers and thumbs out as much as possible. Repeat 2 times.

Chest stretch

Stand straight with your hands on your hips. Bring your elbows back, keeping your shoulders down. Get your elbows as close together as you can comfortably. Hold for 10 seconds and repeat three times. You should feel a stretch across your chest and/or shoulders.

Neck stretch

Pull the chin in slowly, trying to make a double chin. Hold for 2-3 seconds and repeat three times.

Shoulder stretch

Shrug your shoulders up toward your ears. Hold for 2-3 seconds, then relax. Repeat 3 times.

Chapter 9. RSI Concerns for Children and Teenagers

1. A Growing Problem

Karen Jacobs, Chair of Ergonomics for Children and Educational Environment for the American Occupational Therapy Association and occupational therapist at Boston University, conducted a study of childhood musculoskeletal injuries from computer use. She describes the problem: "Computer-related discomfort in childhood and adolescence is of particular concern as the musculoskeletal system and posture are still developing...Young children worldwide are starting to complain now more than ever of musculoskeletal discomfort..." The point to remember is that because the heavy use of electronics starting at a young age is a new enough phenomenon , we don't know the long-term consequences. We do know that the consequences of early repetitive injuries can show up decades later, as the following story illustrates.

RSI-sufferer's story: I worked in a greenhouse as a teenager. I carried bales of peat moss and mixed heavy batches of potting soil and shovelled it into bins. I was proud to be able to do such hard work, and would never think of saying it was too much for me. The next year I couldn't go back because my back and shoulder hurt. Now, decades later, I can't do a lot of the things I love because of my back and shoulder. I can't go backpacking, can't lift my bags of groceries, can't garden. Swimming used to help my back, but I can't do the crawl anymore because of my shoulder and I can't do the breaststroke because that hurts my back. It's like a vicious cycle, limiting my life more and more...all because I was careless when I was 16.

The problem of RSIs amongst youths is not limited to computer use. Game consoles, cell phones, and other gadgets put children at risk for injury. Kids get so involved in their games and projects that it's hard to tear them away from their electronics. An 11-year old boy in Scotland developed tendonitis from spending long periods of time on a Nintendo Gameboy, a condition half-jokingly called "Nintendonitis." Some students have so much pain and disability in their arms and hands that they cannot write their GCSE and A-level exam papers.

Chapter 9. RSI Concerns for Children and Teenagers

Surveys by the Pew Research Centre show that texting by teens is rising sharply. Between 2006 and 2009, the percent of U.S. teens who sent texts rose from 51 percent to 72 percent, an increase of nearly 50 percent in just three years. Half of teens send 50 or more texts *per day*, or 1,500 a month. Overall, girls send nearly three times more texts than boys. One-third of teens age 14-17 send over 100 a day (a practice called hyper-texting), for a whopping 3,000 texts per month. One U.S. teen sent over 9,000 text messages in one month!

The Chartered Society of Physiotherapy (CSP) in the UK warns that unless teens limit their texting they are likely to develop text message

> **My arms hurt so much I'm not gonna make the dance show this year.**

injury (TMI), which the organisation describes as pain and swelling of the tendons at the base of the wrist and thumb, which could create long-term injuries. Other research suggests that the more students text, the more pain they have in their shoulders and necks. (Makes you wonder about the necks, wrists, and shoulders of the competitors in the annual U.S. National Texting Championship sponsored by phone maker LG!)

Other concerns about excessive use of electronic media by children and teens, including loss of social skills and language skills, are beyond the scope of this book, but worth a quick mention. Parents and researchers have observed unexpected awkwardness in face-to-face communication among heavy texters. As one anti-texting teen commented about texting, "It's *so* impersonal." Common use of texting language (acronyms and emoticons) is affecting young people's ability to write grammatically. Surveys show that many teens say that if they could not text they would not communicate at all. Parents are also concerned about their children's exposure to inappropriate content via the Internet. The consequences of texting whilst driving can be deadly for the teens themselves and for other motorists.

Also worth noting but beyond the scope of this book is "toasted skin syndrome" or "laptop thigh" due to sitting with a hot laptop in the lap. The heat can cause mottling on young skin, and can lead to permanent darkening of the skin. Elevated scrotum temperatures, which can reduce sperm production and possibly lead to infertility, have been found in male laptop users.

2. Computers in Schools

According to Dr. Leon Straker of Australia's Curtin University of Technology School of Physiotherapy, nearly 90 percent of children enrolled in school in the U.S. use a computer at school and 60 percent of children in Australia who use laptops in school experience discomfort. He is concerned that back, neck, and shoulder pain amongst young computer users will develop into RSIs as the children mature.

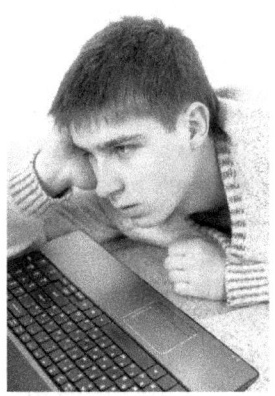

Typical wrong posture of teen laptop user

During its tour of schools in England the Body Action Campaign found the "vast majority using tables which cannot accommodate the range of pupil sizes, plastic bucket chairs and children with their legs dangling, shoulders hunched, without back support and head back gazing up at the screen." Researchers at Cornell University found that the computer equipment used by 40 percent of the U.S. school children they surveyed put the children at risk for postural problems in the future.

When providing computers for students, schools typically place the computers on existing desks, without considering proper workstation design or risks for RSIs. Schools that cannot afford new adjustable ergonomic furniture can adapt what they already have to make the

Chapter 9. RSI Concerns for Children and Teenagers

users safe and comfortable. They can use stacks of books or reams of paper to elevate monitors and cardboard boxes or wooden blocks as footrests. Rolled up towels, jackets, or small pillows can provide lumbar support if they are anchored in place so they don't fall when the child moves around. Simple accessories such as these can be used to adjust the workstations to fit the wide-ranging sizes of elementary school children and promote sensible postures.

Where children use laptop computers at school they should be given external keyboards and mice. The external equipment will compensate for the lack of adjustability of laptops and make it easier for children to position themselves properly, without bending the wrists or holding the head forward.

> **I planned to go to university on a tennis scholarship, but not anymore. My parents have spent so much money on my medical bills I don't know how I can afford to go at all.**

Schools have the opportunity to teach children good computer work habits--habits that can help them avoid RSIs throughout their lives. It's hard to change habits later in life, so it's important to reach kids early. At a minimum, schoolchildren should be taught to:

- Support their feet and lower back.
- Lower their shoulders and relax their arms.
- Keep their elbows level with the keyboard.
- Keep their hands and wrists straight.
- Bend their neck just slightly.
- Keep their eyes level with the top of the screen.

CERGOS, Computer Ergonomics for Elementary School, has information and training activities for children and teachers at http://www.orosha.org/cergos/.

3. Computer Workstation Setup for Young People

Computer workstations for young people are not simply smaller versions of workstations for adults. Computer workstations should adapt to fit a range of sizes, because children change their shapes and sizes as they grow.

Desk Surface

The desk surface needs to be large enough for the keyboard and monitor to be side by side in front of the child.

The surface must be the right height so the child's wrists are straight with the elbows bent at about 90 degrees and the arms relaxed when keying. An adjustable height desk can keep up with a growing child and can be used by other people. Adjustable and sit/stand workstations make it easy for children to change positions.

Monitor

Place the monitor so the top is at or slightly below the child's eye level, directly in front of the child and about an arm's length away. Children should not have to bend their necks to look at their monitors. To avoid eyestrain, the image should be clear and stable and glare should be minimised by placing the monitor perpendicular to the window or using a glare screen.

Keyboard

Place the keyboard straight in front of the child, but away from the front edge of the desk to allow room for forearm support. Thin keyboards are better for children. For smaller children use keyboards without numeric keypads. The keyboard and mouse should be a little below elbow height.

Mouse

Place the mouse close to the keyboard; the child should not have to extend his or her arm to reach the mouse. A mouse bridge, which supports the mouse over the keypad, helps to keep the mouse closer.

Chapter 9. RSI Concerns for Children and Teenagers

The mouse should fit the child's hand; use child-sized mice for smaller children.

Chair

If the chair and work surface are not height adjustable the chair needs to be changed to place the child at the proper height, that is, so hands and wrists are straight, the elbow is bent at 90 degrees, and the eyes are at or just below the top of the monitor.

The chair should allow the child's feet to rest flat on the floor. Otherwise, a footrest is needed. The chair should not have armrests.

Lumbar support, if there is any, needs to fit the small of the child's back.

What do you think about the workstation below?

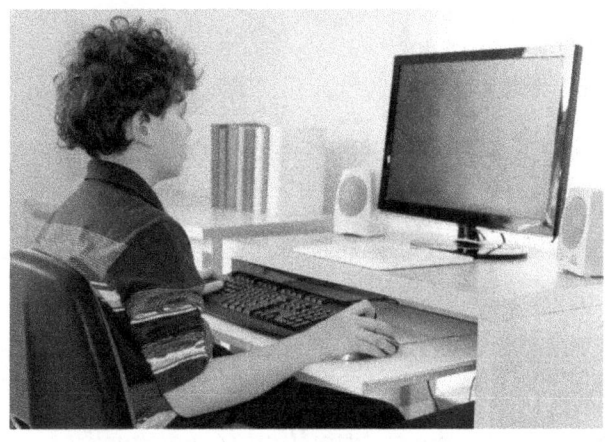

Good: Mouse close to keyboard, separate keyboard surface

Bad: Edge of desk cutting into wrist, glare on screen, monitor too far back.

Improvements: Pad the edges of the keyboard surface. Raise the chair

Chapter 9. RSI Concerns for Children and Teenagers

so that the elbows are closer to right angle (90 degrees). Raising the chair will also avoid resting arms on the desk, will improve hand position, and will move eyesight closer to the top of the screen. Add an anti- glare screen. Move monitor forward and closer to the child.

4. Laptops for Kids

Laptops should be used with a detached keyboard and mouse to allow children to position themselves reasonably.

Laptops should be carried in lightweight two-strap rucksacks instead of hanging off one shoulder. Rolled carrying cases are also good, but most young people don't like them.

Families may be able to modify adult-sized computer setups for young children. Another option is to buy kid-size monitors, keyboards, mice, and chairs. The following are among a growing number of companies that carry computer keyboards, mice, and furniture designed especially for children:

- Ask Ergo Works, Inc.
  www.askergoworks.com/cart_ergo_kids.asp

- Chester Creek Technologies. www.chestercreektech.com

- Tiny Einsteins Computer Products.
  http://www.tinyeinsteins.com/kids_computer_products.html

- QWERTY Keyboard, Computer Keyboards for Children.
  http://www.qwertykeyboard.org/computer-keyboards-for-children

- Source 1 Ergonomics. http://source1ergonomics.com/

5. Safer Computer Practices for Children

A well arranged workstation is important, but it's not enough to prevent RSIs amongst children. Young people should know what they have to do to keep themselves safe. As Karen Jacobs, Boston University physical therapist, said, "As kids embrace technology at a very young age, parents need to not only monitor technology use but instil best-

Chapter 9. RSI Concerns for Children and Teenagers

practices so they are stretching and exercising certain muscles to prevent physical problems in the future."

Posture is an important part of safe computer use. To keep soft tissue healthy, the child should be able to change position easily. A well set up workstation will allow for a range of reasonable postures.

A reasonable posture for a child using a computer looks like this:

- Wrists are relaxed, with the hands and wrists in a straight line (the neutral position). The wrists are not bent back or forward or to the left or the right.
- Legs are at about at about 90 degrees (a right angle) to the spine.
- Knees are even with hips.
- Feet are supported, not dangling.
- Chin is tucked in, eyes are looking straight ahead at the monitor.
- Shoulders are relaxed.
- Elbows are next to body, bent 70-135 degrees, and at almost the same height as the keyboard.

Workers are protected by safety and health regulations, but these regulations do not apply to school children. At school there are some oversight and limitations on computer use, but this is often not the case at home. Computer use is more difficult to control at home than at school, and parents play an important role in doing so. The stakes are very high, because poor computer habits in childhood and adolescence can lead to disability and despair in adulthood.

Following are suggestions to guide parents in their supervision of their children's computer use.

- Limit sedentary screen-based activities to a maximum of two hours a day. This includes computers, video games, television, and texting.

Chapter 9. RSI Concerns for Children and Teenagers

- Require children to take breaks every 20-30 minutes. For breaks to be useful, children need to get up and move around, not merely move to another sedentary activity.

- Teach children the symptoms of RSIs, such as numbness, tingling, soreness, aches, or pains. Make sure they know to tell you right away if they have any problems. Young children may ignore or not be aware of symptoms, so look out for non-verbal cues, like complaints of headaches, avoiding physical activities they used to enjoy, or rubbing their hands, arms, or necks. If you think your child is experiencing any signs of repetitive strain injury, stop their computer use immediately and see a doctor as soon as possible.

- Explain how they can (and why they should) vary tasks, mixing sedentary and non-sedentary activities.

- Teach children to touch type using minimal force, rather than pounding at the keys. This can be done through the use of children's learning CD's.

- Show children how to use keyboard shortcuts and keystrokes instead of a mouse whenever possible.

- Look for ways in which children can reduce their use of computers and other media technology. Encourage them to go to the library and do research with books. Suggest that they call friends or visit them instead of e-mailing or texting. Encourage fun physical activity instead of video games.

- Staying strong and healthy overall guards against RSIs. Make sure children get plenty of regular physical activity, drink water throughout the day, and eat healthy food.

- Take children for regular eye exams. The National Eye Institute in the U.S. reports that children are being diagnosed with nearsightedness more often and at an earlier age because of the amount of time they spend looking at screens.

-

Chapter 9. RSI Concerns for Children and Teenagers

6. Workstation Detectives

Children and teenagers can be taught to assess their own and each other's workstations. They can detect any problems and brainstorm practical solutions that will allow them to position themselves properly and be comfortable at their computers.

Here are questions young people can ask about their computer workstations, whether at home or at school, along with simple, low-cost solutions:

- Are you hunched up or twisted when working at your computer? If yes, re-arrange your work surface so you can position yourself right in front of the monitor.

- Is their enough space under the work surface for your legs and thighs to be comfortable? If not, clear out the space under the desk or use a table for a work surface.

- Are your feet flat on the floor when you are in your chair? If not, use a footrest.

- Is the monitor straight in front of you and about 60 cm away from you? If not, re-position the monitor.

- Is there glare on the monitor? If there is, move it so it is perpendicular to the window and/or add an anti-glare screen.

- Do your eyes line up with screen without bending your neck? If not, raise the monitor on books or blocks or sit on books or pillows.

- Is your mouse close to your keyboard? If not, clear off clutter and put the mouse as close to your keyboard as you can.

- Are your hands and wrists straight when you are keying? If not, raise your chair or raise or lower your work surface.

7. Stretches for Young Computer Users

The American Chiropractic Association recommends frequent breaks with stretches such as the following for young computer users.

Hand circles

Chapter 9. RSI Concerns for Children and Teenagers

Clench hands into fists and move them in circles inward and 10 circles outward—10 times inward and 10 times outward/

Hand squeeze

Place hands in the prayer position and squeeze them together for 10 seconds. Then point them downward and squeeze them together for 10 seconds.

Finger spread

Spread fingers apart and then close them one by one.

Wrap and twist

Stand and wrap arms around the body, then turn all the way to the left and then all the way to the right.

ErgoCoach is break and posture reminder software for children, with animated stretching exercises.
http://magnitudetechnology.com/productshome.asp

> **My dad says no more xbox and no more football. I have to save what's left of my hands for school.**

8. Safer Use of Electronic Gadgets

Electronic gadgets have their own hazards and risks for young people. One video game player described his painful experience: *"It's been hurting for like 4 months now. I am only 19 and I have the thumbs of a 60 year old...Got it from playing too much xbox..."* And here's a similar posted on Twitter: *"...got repetitive strain injury in my wrist from hardcore gaming Spyro. I regret nothing."*

Chapter 9. RSI Concerns for Children and Teenagers

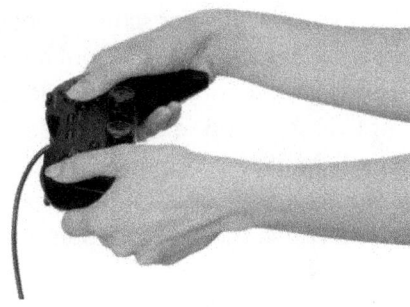

Teen operating game console. Note bent wrists and use of thumbs.

The 2010 winner of the U.S. national teen texting championship couldn't compete this year because of sore wrists. You shouldn't have to give up your gadgets to avoid injury. Here are ways to electronic devices and stay safe:

- Limit the amount of time young people spend on electronic gadgets. CSP recommends limiting texting sessions to 10 minutes at a time.

- Spread the load by alternating fingers and hands when operating gadgets, including texting.

- Avoid bending the neck back to look at game consoles.

- Take frequent breaks to stretch and move around.

- For children, use cell phones sized for small hands.

- Buy cell phones for teens and young children that have parental controls that allow parents to limit calls and/or texting or that only allow a few pre-programmed voice calls. All phones for children and teens should have emergency call buttons and locator buttons.

Firefly (http://www.fireflymobile.com/) and Teddyfone (http://www.kiddyfone.com/) sell mobile phones designed for children.

Sprint Guardian is a bundled app service for Sprint. For customers on

Chapter 9. RSI Concerns for Children and Teenagers

the family plan who use Android phones. Parents can lock their children's cell phones on demand or schedule locks for certain times of the day, such as during dinner, during school hours, and after bedtime. Guardian lets parents limit texting by their children and allows them to see the texts their kids send and receive. The service also has a locator tool. The "Drive First" feature automatically locks a teen's cell phone at speeds over 1.6 kilometres per hour (10 miles per hour). Sprint Guardian is a new service in the United States which is likely to prompt similar services elsewhere.

9. Teens at Work

About 80 percent of U.S. teens work some time during their school years. In the USA, teenage workers get injured at a higher rate than adult workers, even though child labour laws prohibit teens from doing some of the most dangerous jobs. In 2010, 20,000 teens got injured on the job, with 88 fatalities. Why is that? The high injury rate is probably due to teens' inexperience combined with their youth. They are new to the world of work and they may not recognize hazards on the job--like the hazards of working at a poorly designed computer station—nor do they know their rights as workers. Also, their youthful energy and desire to appear like adults may cause them to take unnecessary risks, to not ask questions and to not report problems. As a result of the current economic downturn there are fewer jobs for teens, so they may be reluctant to complain and risk losing their jobs.

Typically, neither school nor workplace prepares teens for working. Most schools do not teach workplace safety and health, and many employers don't provide the extra training and supervision teens need to do their jobs safely.

The National Institute for Occupational Safety and Health, or NIOSH, (http://www.cdc.gov/niosh/topics/youth/) has developed training materials and curricula for teaching youth about workplace safety and health. In keeping with teens' preferred method of learning, the NIOSH materials are visually engaging and specific to different industries. The materials address computer safety, as office work is a typical teen job.

Chapter 10. RSIs in the Workplace

1. Extent of Workplace RSIs and Benefits of Prevention

RSIs are amongst the most common form of work-related disability. According to the Labour Force Survey, 198,000 workers in Great Britain suffered work-related RSIs in 2010/11. That's plenty of reason right there for employers to do everything they can to reduce or eliminate RSIs. The truth is that everyone benefits when employers take steps to prevent RSIs in the workplace. Here's how.

a) Employers

- Retain valued employees.

- Avoid recruitment costs if injured employees cannot return to work (which typically equal one year's salary).

- Avoid training costs for new employees or temporary replacements or for cross-training existing employees.

- Reduce the possibility of more RSIs amongst employees who are covering for injured employees on sick leave.

- Reduce sick pay and insurance/compensation costs.

- Reduce their risk of litigation.

- Maintain workplace morale. The entire workplace suffers when a fellow worker gets injured on the job. Workers perceive a lack of control over the causes of RSIs and perhaps a lack of employer concern for their wellbeing.

- Keep their businesses productive.

- Get a reputation for workplaces that care about their employees.

- Maintain a positive public image. Media information about injuries, citations, and fines can negatively affect public perception (and therefore patronage) of a business.

- Meet their legal responsibilities.

- Help employees lead better lives.

b) Workers
- Retain financial independence.

- Enjoy opportunities for advancement.

- Avoid pain and suffering.

- Maintain their lifestyles and relationships.

- Maintain their self-esteem.

c) Society
- Saves money that can be spent better elsewhere.

- Has plenty of people able to contribute to the community.

RSI-sufferer's story: Amongst staff involved in taking copies in the newsroom of a newspaper, prolonged computer work resulted in RSIs and sickness absence. The company installed better display screen equipment and instituted a break schedule. The cost of the intervention was £47,000. With reduced sickness due to RSIs the payback period was less than 28 months (based on the elimination of three RSIs a year at a cost of £7,749 per RSI). In addition to the financial advantages and reduced risk of RSI, morale improved. Source: HSE

2. Duties on Employers

Employers must follow safety and health regulations. They have a general responsibility to ensure the safety and health of work and take reasonable measures to control risks. They must:

- Appoint a competent person to help meet their health and safety responsibilities.

- Write a health and safety policy for the business.

- Assess the risks.

- Work with health and safety representatives to protect employees.

Chapter 10. RSIs in the Workplace

- Display the HSE-approved health and safety law poster or give each worker the leaflet equivalent to the poster.

- Tell employees about the risks in language they can understand.

- Provide health and safety training.

- Provide any equipment and protective clothing their employees need, at no charge to the employees.

- Provide toilets, washing facilities and safe drinking water.

- Provide adequate first aid supplies, including, at a minimum: a stocked first-aid box and a person appointed to take charge of first aid. Employers must inform all employees about the first aid system they have in place;

- Have insurance that covers employees who get ill or hurt from work and display a copy (electronic or hard copy) of the insurance certificate where workers can easily read it.

- Keep an accident book if you have 10 or more employees (required under social security law).

- Coordinate with other contractors or employers that share the workplace or provide agency workers to protect the health and safety of everyone.

- Report major injuries and deaths at work to the HSE Incident Contact Centre at 0845 300 9923.

- Report other injuries, illnesses, and dangerous incidents at www.hse.gov.uk.

3. Rights and Responsibilities of Employees

Employees have the right to work in environments where health and safety risks are properly controlled. Employers are responsible for controlling those work-related health and safety risks, as discussed above.

Chapter 10.   RSIs in the Workplace

Workers have the right to be provided with safety equipment free of charge. As a worker you can stop work and leave your work area without being disciplined if you have reasonable concerns about your safety. You have the right to have rest breaks during the day, time off from work during the work week, and an annual paid holiday.

Workers who are unable to work because of work-related RSIs may qualify for Industrial Injuries Disablement Benefits (IIDB). Benefits are paid whether or not the person is still working. The amount of the benefit is based on the age of the employee and the severity and longevity of the injury or illness. Directgov (http://www.direct.gov.uk) has more information on IIDB and how to apply for benefits.

Workers also have the right to make injury claims against their employers if they believe their repetitive strain injuries resulted from their jobs.

- In 2002, a court ordered Barclays Bank to pay £244,000 to a former employee who had to give up work at the age of 28 because of pain in her right hand. [The worker] had worked as a bank clerk, and argued that a defective workstation caused her to perform keyboard work in an unsuitable posture. Her symptoms developed over two years, after which time [she] was unable to tie her shoes or even comb her hair.

- A personal assistant was awarded £40,062 for work-related bilateral (both hands) carpal tunnel syndrome and cervical spondylosis. The personal assistant spent 80 percent of her time typing documents with inadequate breaks in order to meet tight deadlines. Plus, the position of her computer monitor required her to turn her head at a 45-degree angle, making her RSIs worse. The court ruled that the employer was in breach of statutory duty by failing to enforce breaks and control the high workload. Claims Management Company www.antriumlegal.com

As a worker you have the right to tell your employer about your safety and health concerns. HSE encourages workers to talk with their supervisors, managers, or safety representatives if they have concerns about their safety work. If that doesn't resolve the problem, you can contact the Environmental Health Department at your local council if you work in an office, shop, restaurant, place of worship, pub, club, nursery, playground, or hotel. If you work for other premises or government offices you should contact the local office of the Health and Safety Executive, which can be found in the telephone book or at http://www.hse.gov.uk/contact/maps/index.htm. It's your right to contact HSE or your local authority if your employer doesn't help you with your safety concerns; your employer is not allowed to discipline you for contacting them.

Workers have health and safety responsibilities too. They must help their employers control risks by:

- Following safety training.

- Paying attention to their own and co-workers' health and safety.

- Cooperating with employers' health and safety programmes.

- Reporting suspected work hazards to the employer, supervisor, or safety representative as soon as possible.

- Reporting injuries as soon as possible.

4. Returning Employees to Work after RSIs

The good news is that the majority of workers who get RSIs will be able to return to work. It may take a while for them to return, and they may need accommodations to do their jobs, but it is to everyone's advantage to help employees return as soon as possible. Workers who are off the job for extended periods of time may suffer depression, isolation, financial insecurity, and difficulty with relationships. The fact is that the longer a worker stays off the job due to injury, illness, or disability, the less likely he or she is ever to return to work.

Returning to work after an RSI is not as simple as it may sound. There's no one-size-fits-all approach; each worker presents a unique situation requiring individual attention. Employers whose employees do repetitive work should have return-to-work systems in place before anyone gets hurt. Employers should tell their employees that it is company policy to help them return to work after an injury or illness. They should also monitor and record all sickness absences, whether

Chapter 10. RSIs in the Workplace

work-related or not. The data collected from monitoring and recording can be used to identify trends and problems in the workplace and correct them to avoid further injuries or illnesses. The Chartered Institute of Personnel and Development (CIPD) offers a free online toolkit to help employers management absences (http://www.cipd.co.uk/hr-resources/practical-tools/absence-management.aspx).

The Statement of Fitness for Work, or fit note, plays an important role in returning to work. From 6 April 2010, the fit note replaces the sick note, or Medical Statement. When a person is unable to work for more than seven days, the doctor writes a fit note, which advises the employer if the employee is "not fit to work," "fit for work" or "may be fit for work."

An employee who "may be fit for work" may be able to return to the job if the employer provides the necessary support. Employer and employee need to work together to implement the suggestions of the doctor. In the fit note the doctor gives information about how the condition will affect the work the employee can do. The doctor may recommend:

- Phased return to work. Gradual increase in work hours, days, or duties;

- Change in work hours. Flexibility to start and/or leave work earlier or later;

- Changes to work duties. For example, more time face-to-face with customers to reduce time on the computer; and/or

- Adaptations to the workplace. For example, providing alternative computer equipment.

If an employer is unable to make the changes an employee needs in order to return to work, the employee cannot return until he or she has recovered more fully. It behoves employers to help employees return to work as quickly as medically advisable. It's better for the business and better for the worker.

RSI-sufferer's story: *"I still can't write, cook, push a pram, kayak or a* *thousand other things but I work full-time (with the help of an understanding employer and voice-activated software-which I am using at the moment). I can also at least play (to some extent) with my children, feed them, and offer some help with childcare. I still have off days, frequently suffer pain but have improved so much."* Source: Watson, M. 2009. Investigating the experiences of people with RSI. http://etheses.qmu.ac.uk/133/

5. Ergonomic Management Programme

"Ergonomics is the scientific discipline concerned with the understanding of the interactions among humans and other elements of a system . . . that applies theory principles, data and methods to design in order to optimize human well-being . . . ergonomists contribute to design and evaluation of tasks, jobs, products, environments and systems in order to make them compatible with the needs, abilities, and limitations of people."— International Ergonomics Association

Ergonomics means fitting the workplace to the worker by modifying or redesigning the job, workstation, tool, or environment. Ergonomics draws from the fields of engineering, and medical and health sciences to optimize the work environment. By identifying ergonomic hazards that can result in an injury or illness, and correcting these hazards, employees can be provided a healthier workplace" Source : www.safety.com

It is much harder to change people than to change furniture, tools and work practices. Ergonomics is a very important concept for reducing work-related RSIs.

The more employees are involved in the ergonomic process, the more successful the process will be. This makes sense because workers are the experts about their jobs; they know more about the hazards and how to correct them than anyone else. Together with managers, supervisors, and health and safety professionals, workers solve problems and take charge of injury prevention.

The United States Occupational Safety and Health Administration, or OSHA, has established guidelines for protecting workers from ergonomic hazards that result in injuries to the musculoskeletal system, including RSIs and other conditions. Whilst each workplace needs to establish its own RSI-prevention programme, the OSHA guidelines provide a framework for those efforts. The following 7-step process is based on OSHA's guidelines.

a) Provide Management Support
Maintaining a safe and healthful workplace where RSI risks are eliminated (or at least reasonably reduced) requires the strong and visible support of top management. Management needs to allocate sufficient resources (finances and personnel). OSHA recommends that employers develop clear goals, assign responsibilities to achieve those goals, provide necessary resources and make sure the designated employees fulfil their responsibilities.

b) Involve Employees
Employees know the most about their jobs and the hazards of their jobs. Ergonomic programmes are much more likely to succeed when employees are involved in significant ways. Employees should be encouraged to voice their concerns and ideas; discuss work methods; participate in the design of work, equipment, procedures, and training; evaluate equipment; and participate in ergonomics task groups.

c) Identify Problems
Organisations need systematic ways to identify RSI hazards. Methods may include reviewing injury and illness records, investigation reports, and insurance claims; interviewing, observing, and surveying employees; conducting risk assessments; and observing workplace conditions.

d) Implement Solutions
Once the problems are known, appropriate solutions can be developed and implemented. Solutions typically involve changes in equipment and/or changes in how the work is done (work practices).

e) Address Reports of Injuries
Management needs to respond promptly to injury reports, making sure employees receive appropriate treatment and follow up, including return-to-work programs. Injury reports and logs can help identify any ongoing RSI problems.

f) Provide Training

Training in ergonomics will make employees, managers and supervisors more effective participants in the ergonomic process ad programme. They also need training in the RSI hazards of the workplace, how to identify them, and what to do in response. Early reporting of RSI symptoms and hazards should be part of training. Studies show that as many as 90 percent of workers do not receive training on RSI risks, symptoms, and safe working procedures.

g) Evaluate Effectiveness of Ergonomic Programme
After the changes have been made, workplaces need to find out whether or not the changes have been effective in eliminating or at least reducing the RSI hazards. Any remaining problems can be dealt with as part of the evaluation.

RSI-sufferer's story. *When editors at a major U.S. newspaper complained about outdated and uncomfortable office equipment, the purchasing manager took the complaints seriously. To make sure the new furniture would make the improvements the editors wanted, the purchasing manger selected employees from every department to try out new equipment. Based on the employees' choices, the purchasing manager bought equipment for employees to test. Chairs were bought first, then keyboard trays, then desks. After the testers had time to "live with" the trial equipment for a reasonable amount of time, the purchasing manager purchased new equipment for all departments based on the testers' recommendations.* Source: HSE

6. Safety in a Weak Economy
When the economy is sluggish employers often look to their safety and health programmes for cutting costs. Most employers find that cutting back on safety to save money comes back to haunt them in the long run. By slashing safety budgets companies risk expensive work injuries and the bad publicity, low morale and production losses that accompany them. They also risk losing other valued workers, because highly skilled workers will look for other jobs if they perceive that their employer are not paying adequate attention to safety. By maintaining a safe working environment companies remain prepared for the eventual economic recovery.

Workers are also endangered by layoffs. With fewer workers on the job each one may be expected to do more work or to work faster. They also may be assigned to jobs for which they are not fully trained or experienced. The heavier workload, faster pace and lack of training are all risk factors for RSIs.

7. Stress on the Job

Improving workstations and work practices addresses the physical hazards of job. That's important, but it's only part of the solution for reducing RSIs. The other part is harder to look at and, perhaps, harder to change. We're talking about the psychosocial aspects of the work environment. "Psychosocial" refers to interactions between people—how well people communicate, get along and support each other. Psychosocial hazards are elements of the workplace--such as management, organisation and environment--that can contribute to physical or psychological harm. A workplace can have the most up-to-date ergonomic equipment and training, but if it doesn't feel good to work there, workers are likely to get hurt. True ergonomics deal with all the factors that make up a workplace physical and psychosocial.

"Psychosocial" and "stress" are two words that often go together. The National Institute for Occupational Safety and Health, or NIOSH, defines workplace stress as: "...the harmful physical and emotional responses that occur when the requirements of the job do not match the capabilities, resources, or needs of the worker. Job stress can lead to poor health and even injury." According to NIOSH workplace stress can cause or aggravate a number of health problems, including musculoskeletal disorders.

There's no doubt that job stress is on the rise worldwide. A survey conducted for the European Agency for Safety and Health at Work (EU-OSHA),found that job-related stress is a concern for the large majority of the European workforce. Seventy-nine percent of the managers surveyed think stress is as important an issue for their companies as accidents.

Stress sets off a "fight or flight" reaction in the brain: the pulse quickens, breathing deepens, and muscles tense up. When the stress resolves, the brain goes back to normal and all is well, but when stress is constant, the body remains in its heightened state, causing undo wear and tear on the body's systems and tissues. Plus, stress is also distracting; it's hard to focus on doing your job safely when you are all wound up.

a) Job Stressors

It's no secret what makes a job stressful:
- High work demand, including long work hours/mandatory overtime
- Tight deadlines
- Shift work
- Lack of family friendly policies
- Bad relationship with supervisor
- Racist, sexists, or bullying supervisor
- Unsafe or unpleasant working conditions, including ergonomic problems
- Lack of co-worker support
- Work that is either too challenging or not challenging enough
- Not being appreciated for your work
- Lack of control over work
- No possibilities for advancement within the organisation
- Dissatisfaction with the job
- Ambiguity about job responsibilities
- Too much or too little responsibility
- Poor communication within the organisation
- Concern about job security from plant closings/layoff/relocation/automation

A stress and musculoskeletal disorder study by HSE found that high exposure to physical and psychosocial risk factors on the job increased the likelihood of reporting musculoskeletal complaints, including neck, should, elbow/forearm, hand/wrist, and back complaints.

b) Reducing Stress

What can be done about job stress? NIOSH finds that recognition of employees for good work performance, opportunities for career development, organisational culture that values individual workers, and management actions that are consistent with the values of the organisation are associated with low-stress and high-productivity workplaces.

Solutions vary with each workplace, and might include:

- Ensuring that the workload is in line with the employees'

abilities.
- Designing jobs that are rewarding and allow workers to use their skills.
- Clearly defining roles and responsibilities.
- Involving employees in decisions that affect their jobs.
- Improving communications.
- Providing opportunities for social interaction amongst employees.
- Establishing flexible work schedules that support employees in meeting their family and personal responsibilities.

Personal factors also play a role in the individual's ability to manage stress. In other words, some people are better able to handle stress than others. For people who turn pressure into stress, decision-making, efficiency and compliance with safety practices can be compromised. So, in addition to making changes in work equipment and physical environment, employers can help reduce stress on the job by providing training on stress management.

c) HSE Management Standards

HSE has developed Management Standards for work-related stress that establishes a process for controlling stress and identifying the characteristics of an organisation where stress is being managed effectively. The approach involves five steps:

1. Identify the risk factors.
2. Determine who can be harmed and how.
3. Evaluate the risks.
4. Record your findings.
5. Monitor and review.

The Management Standards address six key areas:

1. **Demand**. Workload, work pattern, work environment.
2. **Control**. What workers have to say about the way they do their work.
3. **Support**. The encouragement and resources provided by the employer, managers, and colleagues.
4. **Relationships**. Promoting positive working to avoid conflicts. Dealing with unacceptable behaviour.

5. **Role**. Whether workers understand their roles and whether the organisation ensures workers do not have conflicting roles.
6. **Change**. How change is managed and communicated in the organisation.

Experts agree that changes to major areas such as these require the participation of everyone involved. It's not enough to marginally involve employees in the solution. As NIOSH puts it: "*Bringing workers and managers together in a committee or problem-solving group may be an especially useful approach for developing a stress prevention program. Research has shown these participatory efforts to be effective in dealing with ergonomic problems in the workplace, partly because they capitalize on workers' firsthand knowledge of hazards encountered in their jobs.*"

The more employees participate in identifying stress reduction needs and developing prevention programs, the more specific the solutions will be for that workplace. The combination of employee engagement and success in reducing stress in the work environment is key to reducing the risks for RSIs.

Chapter 11. Relevant Regulations

Many countries have regulations governing the use of computers in the workplace. It is impossible to list the regulations for all countries; so following are key regulations from the UK and the USA. In addition to national regulations, localities may have their own rules for safe computer use. Laws and regulations change all the time so the information below is correct at the time of print but might change.

1. Great Britain

a) Health and Safety at Work Act (HASAW)
Primary regulation concerning occupational safety and health in the UK. Employers must assess risks to their employees and other people who might be affected by what they do, such as children or the public. They must take reasonable steps to minimise the risks. In addition, employers must protect employees after they return to work if they are more vulnerable to risks because of injury, illness, or disability.

b) Workplace (Health, Safety, & Welfare) Regulations
Applies to most workplaces (except those involving construction works on construction sites, in or on ships, or below ground at a mine) and covers a number of basic health, safety, and welfare issues.

c) Health and Safety (Display Screen Equipment) Rules
Employers who have employees who habitually use display screen equipment (DSE) as a significant part of their normal work must:

- Analyse workstations to assess and reduce risks. Employers must look at the whole workstation, including equipment, furniture, and the work environment. They must also look at the task being done and any special needs of the individual employee. Employers should assess workstations when a new workstation is set up, when a new user starts work, or when a major change is made to an existing workstation or to the use of the workstation.

- Ensure workstations meet specified minimum requirements covering chairs, lighting, screens, keyboards, desks, software, and the work environment.

- Plan work activities to include breaks or changes of activity depending on the nature of the activity. The law does not specify the number or length of breaks.

- Provide eye and eyesight tests on request by employees who habitually use DSE as a significant part of their normal day-to-day work. The employer must pay for spectacles if special corrective spectacles are required for DSE work. The employer does not have to pay for normal spectacles.

- Provide health and safety information and training on how to use their workstations safely to avoid health problems. The employer must also provide information on computer use health and safety and on what the employer is doing to comply with the regulation. Topics should include posture, adjusting furniture, desk organisation, adjusting screens and lighting to avoid reflections and glare, breaks and changes of activity, risk assessments, how to apply for an eye test and how to report problems about their work.

An IT Assessments Officer was awarded £2,750 in injury compensation for having developed tenosynovitis in the right wrist at work. The employer conceded it had breached sections of the Health and Safety (Display Screen Equipment) Regulations.

d) Disability Discrimination Act (DDA)
Employers must make reasonable adjustments to disabled employees' work to make sure they are not treated less favourably than other employees.

e) Reporting Regulations
Under the Reporting of Injuries, Diseases and Dangerous Occurrences Regulations (RIDDOR), employers, the self-employed and people in control of work premises are required to report serious workplace accidents, occupational diseases and close calls. RSIs are reportable if they lead to a major injury or result in absence lasting more than three working days.

Chapter 11. Relevant Regulations

f) Employee Rights Act
Employers must adopt fair procedures before dismissing an employee for being absent from work due to sickness.

g) Provision and Use of Work Equipment Regulations
Employers must assess and prevent or control health and safety risks from equipment they use at work.

h) Data Protection Act
Employers must keep certain sickness absence data.

i) Management of Health & Safety at Work Regulations
Employers must assess risks that arise from work activities, including people who are not in their employment but may be affected by the work. Affected people may include children who are affected by work at their school, the general public or others.

j) Employment Act (Dispute Resolution)
Employers must adopt minimum discipline, dismissal, and grievance procedures.

k) Employers Liability (Compulsory Insurance) Act
Most UK employers are required to purchase Employers Liability Insurance, which covers injuries, illnesses, harassment, bullying, discrimination, unfair dismissal, work-related stress and workplace violence. It is up to the employee to show that the employer has a legal obligation to provide compensation.

2. United States

a) Occupational Safety and Health Act of 1974
Under the Occupational Safety and Health Act of 1974 (OSH Act), employers must provide employees with work and places of work that are free from recognized hazards that could cause serious harm. This is called the General Duty Clause.

Whilst some states have adopted ergonomics regulations, there is no ergonomics law for the entire country. The Occupational Safety and Health Administration (OSHA) has issued voluntary ergonomics guidelines. In the absence of a specific regulation, OSHA uses the General Duty Clause to cite and fine employers who risk ergonomic injuries to employees. OSHA has been issuing citations for ergonomic hazards since 2003.

b) Fair Labour Standards Act (FLSA)
Amongst other provisions, FLSA sets minimum standards for youth employment, addressing the hours teens can work and the type of work they can do. Many states have more stringent child labour laws as well as laws requiring breaks.

c) Workers' Compensation Laws
Most employers in the United States are required to purchase workers' compensation insurance, which pays medical costs and indemnity for employees who are injured or made ill on the job. All states have workers' compensation laws, which are administered by the states and differ from state to state. Workers' compensation insurance protects employers from legal action by employees who have been injured or made ill as a result of their work.

d) Whistleblower Protections
Whistleblower protection laws protect people (including workers) who report unsafe working conditions. In 2012, the U.S. Department of Labour fined a railroad more than $300,000 for firing an employee for reporting a work-related injury.

e) Americans with Disabilities Act (ADA)
Prohibits discrimination on the basis of employment, State and local government, public accommodations, commercial facilities, transportation and telecommunications.

Claims Management Company www.antriumlegal.com

Chapter 13. Stretchers and Exercises

Chapter 12. Conclusion

You've read it all, you've read the sufferer's stories. Surely you do NOT want to be one of these sufferers. You don't need to be.

Therefore you MUST pay attention to your own health. Your office environment, your mobile phone, your game console, your laptop are NOT safe for your health unless YOU make them safe by taking breaks and doing regular exercises.

In my opinion, all electronic devices from this modern society should have pop-up software on that throws messages at the user like "get off this computer" or " stop texting" or " time for exercises" or "put me down".

I have break-software on my computer and I urge everybody to do the same. The software I use is: www.breakremindersoftware.com **(only available for PC, not for Mac**) and in my opinion this should be installed on each computer that is sold anywhere in the world. The software monitors the time you work on the computer and it alerts you when you need to take a break. You can set it to block your keyboard during breaks so you cannot work. You can choose to override your settings should you wish to do so but I suggest you set them as "Whatever I do, give me a break". My settings are as follows:

- I have a break for 20 seconds every 10 minutes and I've set the software so that my keyboard is blocked. Therefore every 10 minutes I do some gentle neck and arm exercises.

- I have a 10-minute break every hour and my software is set so my keyboard is blocked, which forces me to get up and do something else for 10 minutes.

If you can afford it, invest in www.breakremindersoftware.com. It is the best piece of software available for an office environment. You have been warned: install it as a matter of urgency if you can afford it.

If you cannot afford it: force yourself to take regular breaks.

Chapter 13. Stretchers and Exercises

I do realise that some of the ergonomic furniture and aids pictured or talked about in this book are expensive but if you can, drink a few cups of coffee less per month or reduce your alcohol consumption and buy some of the aids to prevent RSI in your life.

I end this book with the message I've put at the beginning:

> **It is no joke, really, please take this seriously and look after your future health.**
>
> **Don't ignore your symptoms as it really comes down to this one simple message:**
>
> **ACT NOW**
>
> **OR**
>
> **SUFFER FOREVER!**

Chapter 13. Stretchers and Exercises

Hopefully you will want to do these exercises on a regular basis. I have listed all the exercises from this book here again so it is convenient for you to refer to them, all together, rather than spread out throughout the book.

1. Stretches for Computer Users
Shoulder Shrug

Raise the top of your shoulders toward your ears until you feel slight tension in your neck and shoulders. Hold for 3-5 seconds. Relax your shoulders and repeat 3 times.

Shoulder Roll 1

Sit down and make yourself as tall as possible. Slowly roll your shoulder to the back in a circular motion. Then roll your shoulders forward. Repeat 5 times each way.

Shoulder Roll 2

Stand up and put your hands at your side and relax your shoulders. Slowly roll your shoulders in a backwards and forewords direction and try to make the circle you make by rolling as large as possible. Repeat 5 times each way.

Shoulder Stretch

Sit down on a chair and put your hands behind your heads with your elbows pointing outwards. Push your elbows gently forward towards each other and try to stretch until the tips of your elbows touch. Hold for 5 seconds and repeat a few times.

Neck Stretcher 1

Drop your head slowly to the left, trying to touch your left shoulder with your left ear until you feel the stretch in the right side of your neck. Hold for 3 seconds Bring your head back to normal position. Drop your head slowly to the right, trying to touch your right shoulder with your right ear until you feel the stretch in the left side of your

Chapter 13. Stretchers and Exercises

neck. Hold for 3 seconds. Bring your head back to normal position. Repeat 3 times each way.

Neck Stretcher 2

Drop your head slowly to the left, trying to touch your left shoulder with your left ear . Then, slowly drop your chin to your chest; turn your head all the way to the left, then all the way to the right. You should feel the stretch in your neck. Repeat 3 times and do the other side.

Neck Stretcher 3

Turn your head sideways as far as comfortable as you are looking to the left. Bend your neck over to look at the floor until you feel a stretch. Hold for 3 seconds. Return your head in original position and do the other side. Repeat 3 times.

Wrist Turns

Sit down and put your arms next to you. Turn your arms and wrist so that your palm faces outwards away from your body and then back inwards. Feel the stretch in your lower arm. Hold for 3 seconds. Repeat 3 times.

Upper Arm Stretcher

Sit down or stand up. Put your right arm forwards with the palm facing the floor. Now put your left hand underneath your right elbow and turn the palm of your right hand facing towards the left. With your left arm pull your right arm towards you so you can feel the stretch in your right upper arm. Hold for 3 seconds. Repeat 3 times with each arm.

Head turns

Drop your head down towards your chest as far as it feels comfortable. Turn your head left trying to look at your left upper arm and hold for 2 seconds. Turn your head right trying to look at your right upper arm and hold for 2 seconds. Repeat 5 times each side.

Chapter 13. Stretchers and Exercises

Back Curl and Leg Stretch

Hold onto your right shin with your right hand. Lift your right leg off the floor. Bend forward, curling your back, and bring your nose toward your knee. Repeat with the other leg.

Leg Stretcher

Sit on a chair and make yourself as tall as possible. Stretch one leg forwards and try to point your toes as far as possible towards you and hold for 5 seconds. You should feel the stretch throughout your whole leg. Repeat with the other leg. Do 3 times for each leg.

Forward lean

Sit on a chair and put your elbows and arms on your thighs and let your hands relax. Lean your head downwards. Sit like that and take 4 to 5 breaths and return in the sitting position.

Trunk Stretcher (the part of your body between your neck and your waist)

Sit on a chair and make yourself as tall as possible. Drop your arms by your side. Move your left hand towards the floor as far as you can but make sure that your trunk stays upright. Hold your arm for 5 seconds. Return to sitting position and repeat with right arm. Repeat with each arms 3 times.

Forearm Twist

Sit down on a chair and put your hands on your lap with the palms facing your legs. Relax your shoulders. Turn your hands so that your palm is now facing up. Gently push your thumbs outwards as far as comfortable and hold for 3 seconds. Turn your hand again to face your legs. Repeat with 5 times.

Stretch your arms and fingers

Sit on a chair and make yourself as tall as possible. Put both of your arms forwards with the palm of your hands facing you. Interlink your fingers. Roll your palms/arms so that they now face away from you.

Chapter 13. Stretchers and Exercises

Stretch by reaching out as far as you can and hold for 5 seconds. Feel the stretch in lower arm and fingers. Repeat 3 times.

Stretch your arms and shoulders

Sit on a chair and make yourself as tall as possible. Put both of your arms forwards with the palm of your hands facing you. Interlink your fingers. Roll your palms/arms so that they now face away from you. Move your arms so they are now above your head. Stretch by reaching out as far as you can and hold for 5 seconds. Repeat 3 times.

Arm Shakes

Sit on a chair, drop your shoulders and let your arms hang loosely next to your body. Shake your arms and hands for 5 seconds. Repeat 5 times.

Ankle Pumps

Sit and put your feet flat on the floor. Lift your foot upwards so only your heel is touching the floor. Hold for 3 seconds. Now, roll your foot forwards, lifting up your heel so only your toes are touching the floor. Hold for 3 seconds. Repeat in both directions 3 times.

2. Stretches for Texters

Thumb stretch

With the right palm facing down, hold the thumb of the right hand with the fingers of the left hand. Pull the thumb gently and hold for 10 seconds. Repeat three times, then reverse hands.

Arm stretch

Stretch your left arm in front of you, palm up. Place your right hand on top of the left with fingers and thumbs lined up. Point your fingers down and hold for 10 seconds. You should feel a gentle stretch on the inside of your left forearm/wrist. Repeat three times, then reverse hands.

Chapter 13. Stretchers and Exercises

Finger stretch

Hold hand out, palm down. Spread fingers and thumbs as far as you can. Hold 2-3 seconds. Then make a fist and hold 2-3 seconds. Repeat 3 times.

Arm and finger stretcher

Sit in a chair and make yourself as tall as possible. Lean back as far as you can so you are looking towards the ceiling. Spread your arms (like you did as a kid when you were flying an aeroplane) and rotate your arms left and right. Spread your fingers and thumbs out as much as possible. Repeat 2 times.

Chest stretch

Stand straight with your hands on your hips. Bring your elbows back, keeping your shoulders down. Get your elbows as close together as you can comfortably. Hold for 10 seconds and repeat three times. You should feel a stretch across your chest and/or shoulders.

Neck stretch

Pull the chin in slowly, trying to make a double chin. Hold for 2-3 seconds and repeat three times.

Shoulder stretch

Shrug your shoulders up toward your ears. Hold for 2-3 seconds, then relax. Repeat 3 times.

3. Stretches for Young Computer Users
Hand circles

Clench hands into fists and move them in circles inward and 10 circles outward—10 times inward and 10 times outward/

Hand squeeze

Place hands in the prayer position and squeeze them together for 10 seconds. Then point them downward and squeeze them together for 10 seconds.

Chapter 13.   Stretchers and Exercises

Finger spread

Spread fingers apart and then close them one by one.

Wrap and twist

Stand and wrap arms around the body, then turn all the way to the left and then all the way to the right.

Vendors of Equipment and Software for RSI Prevention

A growing number of manufacturers produce ergonomically designed equipment. The following list of vendors represent only a small percentage of those that sell software and equipment that can help prevent RSIs and improve conditions for those recovering from repetitive strain injuries.

Inclusion in this list or in the text of this book does not indicate endorsement of products or vendors, nor does absence from the list indicate lack of approval. Many products billed as ergonomically designed are not effective in preventing RSIs; buyers need to study the products carefully to see if they meet their needs.

Software

Break Reminder Software

www.breakremindersoftware.com

www.workpace.com

www.rsiprevention.com

www.rsiguard.com

Equipment

Alternative Workstations

Anthro (www.Anthro.com)

Ergo Desk (www.ErgoDesk.com)

Ergolcd.com (http://www.ergolcd.com/)

Ergotron (www.ergotron.com)

GeekDesk (www.geekdesk.com/)

Nielsen http://www.nielsen-associates.co.uk/sit-stand

Steelcase (http://www.steelcase.com)

Treadmill Desk (www.treadmill-desk.com/)

Alternative Keyboards

ErgonomicKeyboards www.ergonomickeyboards.org

FrogPad www.frogpad.com

Keytools www.keytools.co.uk/keyboards

Source 1 Ergonomics. www.source1ergonomics.com

Alternative Mice and Other Pointing Devices

Amazon.com www.amazon.co.uk/Foot-Mouse-Slipper-Programmable-Pedal/dp/B0061DVAOK

FrogPad (www.frogpad.com)

Gizmag www.gizmag.com

Keytools www.keytools.com/mice

Liberator www.liberator.co.uk/headmouse-extreme.html

Price Selector (http://uk.price-selector.net/search/foot%20pedal%20mouse?campid=5336926831)

Source 1 Ergonomics http://www.source1ergonomics.com

Techcess http://www.techcess.co.uk/5_1_headmouse.php

The Human Solution www.thehumansolution.com/mice.html

Workstation Equipment for Children

Ask Ergo Works, Inc.http://www.askergoworks.com

Chester Creek Technologies http://www.chestercreektech.com

Tiny Einsteins Computer Products http://www.tinyeinsteins.com

QWERTY Keyboard, Computer Keyboards for Children www.qwertykeyboard.org

Published by IMB Publishing 2015

Copyright and Trademarks: This publication is Copyrighted 2015 by IMB Publishing. All products, publications, software and services mentioned and recommended in this publication are protected by trademarks. In such instance, all trademarks & copyright belong to the respective owners. All rights reserved. No part of this book may be reproduced or transferred in any form or by any means, graphic, electronic, or mechanical, including photocopying, recording, taping, or by any information storage retrieval system, without the written permission of the authors. Pictures used in this book are either royalty free pictures bought from stock-photo websites or have the source mentioned underneath the picture.

Disclaimer and Legal Notice: This product is not legal or medical advice and should not be interpreted in that manner. You need to do your own due-diligence to determine if the content of this product is right for you. The authors and the affiliates of this product are not liable for any damages or losses associated with the content in this product. While every attempt has been made to verify the information shared in this publication, neither the author nor the affiliates assume any responsibility for errors, omissions or contrary interpretation of the subject matter herein. Any perceived slights to any specific person(s) or organization(s) are purely unintentional. We have no control over the nature, content and availability of the web sites listed in this book.

The inclusion of any web site links does not necessarily imply a recommendation or endorse the views expressed within them. IMB Publishing takes no responsibility for, and will not be liable for, the websites being temporarily unavailable or being removed from the Internet.

The accuracy and completeness of information provided herein and opinions stated herein are not guaranteed or warranted to produce any particular results, and the advice and strategies, contained herein may not be suitable for every individual. The author shall not be liable for any loss incurred as a consequence of the use and application, directly or indirectly, of any information presented in this work. This publication is designed to provide information in regard to the subject matter covered.

The information included in this book has been compiled to give an overview of the subject and detail some of the symptoms, treatments etc. that are available. It is not intended to give medical advice. For a firm diagnosis of any health condition, and for a treatment plan suitable for you and your dog, you should consult your veterinarian or consultant.

The writer of this book and the publisher are not responsible for any damages or negative consequences following any of the treatments or methods highlighted in this book. Website links are for informational purposes and should not be seen as a personal endorsement; the same applies to the products detailed in this book. The reader should also be aware that although the web links included were correct at the time of writing, they may become out of date in the future.

www.ingramcontent.com/pod-product-compliance
Lightning Source LLC
Chambersburg PA
CBHW060836050426
42453CB00008B/719